High-Resolution Electrophoresis and Immunofixation

High-Resolution Electrophoresis and Immunofixation

Techniques and Interpretation

David F. Keren, M.D.
Associate Professor of Pathology, Microbiology, and Immunology
Head, Biochemistry Section, and
Director, Clinical Immunology Laboratory
Department of Pathology
The University of Michigan Medical School

Butterworths
Boston London Durban Singapore Sydney Toronto Wellington

Every effort has been made to ensure that the drug dosage schedules
within this text are accurate and conform to standards accepted at
time of publication. However, as treatment recommendations vary in
the light of continuing research and clinical experience, the reader is
advised to verify drug dosage schedules herein with information found
on product information sheets. This is especially true in cases of new
or infrequently used drugs.

Library of Congress Cataloging-in-Publication Data

Keren, David F.
   High resolution electrophoresis and immunofixation.

   Includes bibliographies and index.
   1. Blood protein disorders—Diagnosis.
2. Blood protein electrophoresis.   3. Immunoelectrophoresis.
4. Immunodiagnosis.   I. Title. [DNLM: 1. Electrophoresis—methods.   2. Immunoelectrophoresis—methods. QU 25 K39h]
RC647.B6K46   1987   616.07´56   86–21591
ISBN 0-409-90021-4

Butterworth Publishers
80 Montvale Avenue
Stoneham, MA 02180

10 9 8 7 6 5 4 3 2 1

Printed in the United States of America

To my family

CONTENTS

PREFACE

The world of clinical laboratory medicine is changing rapidly. At the same time that basic science is providing us with a great variety of techniques that are helpful and sometimes essential for understanding disease, society demands responsibility from the laboratory for using only those techniques that are proven to be of diagnostic utility. Under these same pressures, we are asked to update our methodologies to take advantage of newer cost-effective procedures for arriving more quickly at the proper diagnosis.

While many laboratories were already making efforts to be efficient, the previous system had no incentive for rewarding the cost-effective laboratory. Today's laboratorian is faced with the difficult task of trying to stay abreast of the most recent *useful* methodologies to provide the patient with state-of-the-art medicine while trying to balance the budget sheet with the laboratory manager.

Fortunately, these goals are not necessarily antagonistic. Indeed, the search for more efficient methodologies and instrumentation often results in techniques with greater overall capabilities. One such happy occurrence is the recent trend toward using high-resolution electrophoresis for diagnosis of protein abnormalities. While many research procedures such as two-dimensional electrophoresis have yet to show their cost-effectiveness in the clinical laboratory, it is clear that high-resolution electrophoresis and immunofixation methodologies can do much to make a faster, more sensitive, and less expensive diagnosis than older methods.

This text is designed to acquaint the reader with the available methodologies and instrumentation for performing high-resolution electrophoresis and immunofixation. A strategy is presented for using these procedures to facilitate the diagnosis of a variety of serum protein abnormalities. Finally, a large number of case examples are presented to illustrate the uses of these new procedures and their possible caveats.

I would like to thank the many people who have helped in development of this material. Special thanks are due to Dr. John Carey, Ms. Anne DiSante, and Ms. Donna Bush for reviewing the text to eliminate some of my more outrageous statements. Ms. Sharon Bordine and Ms. Linda Thomas were extremely helpful in providing additional information about specific cases. Drs. Fred Holtz and Richard Lash initiated the development of immunofixation in our laboratory. Last and by no means least, I am indebted to the technologists in our Clinical Immunology Laboratory for their superb efforts in providing the quality samples used to illustrate this text, to Mr. Craig Biddle and Mr. Eddie Burke for their photographic skills, Ms. Robin Kunkel for illustrations, and to our pathology residents at the University of Michigan for keeping me honest by always asking "why?"

D.F.K.

CHAPTER 1

Methods and Rationale for High-Resolution Electrophoresis

REVIEW OF PROTEIN STRUCTURE AND ELECTROPHORETIC TECHNIQUES

The term "electrophoresis" refers to the migration of charged particles in an electrical field. Modern versions of this technique to determine the migration and concentration of proteins from serum, urine, and cerebrospinal fluid, and their clinical relevance, are reviewed in this volume. The success of electrophoresis in separating serum proteins into clinically useful fractions results from the heterogeneity of the charges of these molecules. It is useful, therefore, to review briefly the structure of these molecules that results in the observed migration.

Protein Structure and Electrophoretic Mobility

Proteins are composed of amino acids; the general structure is shown in Figure 1-1. The R groups attached to the alpha carbon can be neutral, acidic, or basic (Table 1-1). When in solution, these amino acids behave as both acids and bases due to the simultaneous presence of at least one carboxyl and one amino group on each amino acid. This results in the formation of a *zwitterion* in aqueous solution, that is, a molecule in which both the amino and carboxyl ends are ionized, yet the molecule is electrically neutral (Figure 1-2). Since this molecule is electrically neutral, that is, *isoelectric,* it would not migrate in an electrical field.

By altering the pH of an aqueous solution, the charge on an amino acid can be changed. In acidic solution, the amino acid accepts a proton on its carboxylate group, resulting in a net positive charge on the molecule (Figure 1-2). The positively charged cation thus formed would migrate toward the negative pole (cathode) in an electrical field. Conversely, in basic solution the ammonium group gives up a proton, leaving the amino acid with a net negative

1

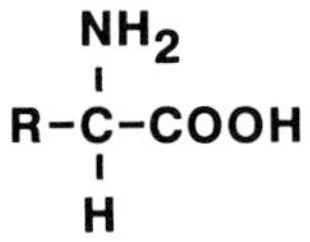

$$\begin{array}{c} NH_2 \\ | \\ R-C-COOH \\ | \\ H \end{array}$$

Figure 1-1.   General structure of amino acids.

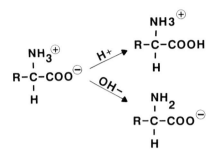

Figure 1-2.   Effect of acidic and basic solutions on amino acid charge.

charge (Figure 1-2). This negatively charged anion now migrates toward the positive pole (anode) in an electrical field. Obviously, the pH of the solution and the nature of the R group (Table 1-1) have an important effect on the migration of individual amino acids.

Proteins and peptides are composed of amino acids that are joined by

Table 1-1   List of Common Amino Acids

	Neutral Amino Acids		
Aliphatic	Aromatic	Sulfur-Containing	Secondary Amino
Glycine	Phenylalaine	Cystine	Proline
Alanine	Tyrosine	Cysteine	Hydroxyproline
Valine	Tryptophan	Methionine	
Leucine			
Isoleucine			
Serine			
Threonine			

	Acidic Amino Acids
	Aspartic Acid
	Glutamic Acid

	Basic Amino Acids
	Histidine
	Arginine
	Lysine
	Hydroxylysine

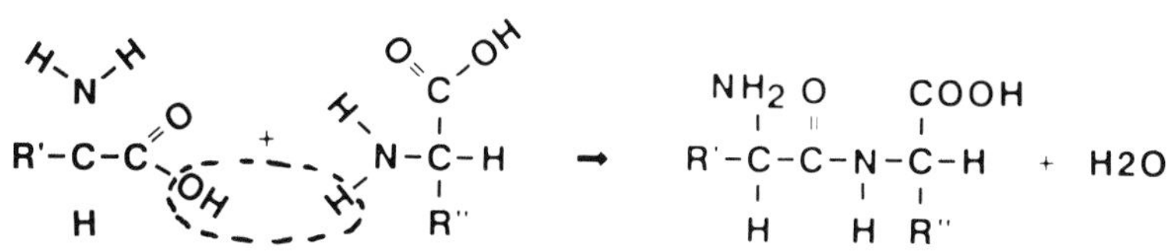

Figure 1-3. Peptide bond formation involves linkage of the carboxyl group of one amino acid with the amino group of another.

peptide bonds, the linkage of the carboxyl group of one amino acid to the amino group of the next. During the process, a water molecule is given off and a peptide bond is produced (Figure 1-3). The resulting molecule has the charge characteristics inherent in the R groups together with the carboxyl and amino terminal groups.

Because the amino acid composition of a given protein is unique, it will have a specific charge and migration pattern under defined conditions during electrophoresis. Protein molecules, like their constituent amino acids, have their overall charge determined by the pH of the solvent; there will be a specific pH at which the negative and positive charges balance and at which the protein will not migrate. The pH at which the positive and negative charges of a given protein balance is referred to as its *isoelectric point* (pI). The pI is constant and highly specific for a given protein molecule.

During electrophoresis, when a protein is dissolved in a solution that is acidic relative to protein pI, it will gain protons and migrate to the cathode. In solutions that are basic relative to protein pI, the protein will donate protons and migrate toward the anode. For proteins in the serum, urine, and cerebrospinal fluid, the amount of charge due to free sulfhydryl groups is negligible with regard to electrophoretic migration. Structures for specific proteins relevant to clinical diagnosis by electrophoresis and immunofixation are considered in the next chapter.

Moving Boundary Electrophoresis

Early studies on the electrophoretic mobilities of proteins, carried out by Tiselius [1], employed a liquid medium. For these studies, Tiselius devised a U-shaped electrophoretic cell and employed a Schlieren band optical system to detect the degree of refraction of light by proteins as they passed through the tube. A specific volume of a protein mixture was dissolved in buffer, and the solution was carefully layered in the electrophoresis tube below the same buffer. The buffer was placed in contact with electrodes, and the sensitive optical band method was used to monitor the progress of protein fractions during electrophoresis.

When the current was turned off at the end of the run, a mixing of the boundaries occurred and only the fractions at the extreme cathodal and anodal ends of the tube could be collected in a relatively purified form. Therefore, originally this moving boundary electrophoresis was often used to test the success of protein purification that had been performed by other means. Although crude by today's standards, such early techniques were sufficiently sensitive to allow Michaelis to determine isoelectric points on the solutions of the marginally purified enzymes he had for study [2]. This moving boundary technique was also instrumental in the original definition of the major fractions of human serum proteins as albumin, alpha-1, alpha-2, beta, and gamma globulin.

Zone Electrophoresis

As stated previously, one of the key practical problems with moving boundary electrophoresis was its inability to achieve a complete separation of electrophoretically adjacent major protein fractions. Also, the refractive index that was used to quantify the proteins in moving boundary electrophoresis was limited in its discrimination of subtle differences. The development of zone electrophoresis made it possible to overcome these difficulties by providing a stable support medium in which proteins could migrate and be stained and quantified. Zone electrophoresis, then, offered the important feature of stabilizing the migration of the proteins, which moving boundary electrophoresis could not achieve.

The first major supporting medium for electrophoresis was filter paper. Studies using this support medium were begun as early as 1939; however, it was not until the early 1950s that these techniques were simplified and rigorously defined for practical use in clinical laboratories.

The use of filter paper as a support medium introduced new variables into electrophoresis. As with the moving boundary technique, the migration of individual proteins depended on pI of the molecule, pH of the buffer, electrolyte concentration of the buffer, and amount of current applied. However, the texture of the filter paper was found to be important, because it offered substantially more resistance to the movement of the proteins than was the case in the free-moving boundary system.

Early in the development of paper electrophoresis, Kunkel and Tiselius [3] observed that the texture of paper products differed and that this resulted in different migration of proteins depending on the brand of paper used. Although the actual distance from the origin that human serum albumin would migrate may be greater on one brand of paper than on another brand, Kunkel and Tiselius observed that the relationship between albumin and the subsequent fractions was constant and could be used to create a correction factor specific for that preparation of filter paper. It was also observed that the migration of smaller molecules was less affected by the type of paper than was the migration of larger molecules [4].

The introduction of paper as a support medium introduced the effect known as *electroosmosis* or *endosmosis* as another factor influencing the migration of proteins. The support medium (filter paper, in the present case, but also cellulose acetate and agar) acquires a negative charge relative to the buffer solution. Obviously, the paper support medium is stationary and cannot migrate; however, the positively charged buffer solution will flow toward the negative electrode (cathode).

Understanding endosmosis is important in relating the migration of proteins to their surface charge. For instance, most systems that are used in the study of human serum, cerebrospinal, or urine proteins use an alkaline buffer with a pH of 8.6. At this pH almost all serum proteins, including the gamma globulins, will have a negative charge. Yet they do not all migrate toward the anode. Most of the gamma globulins and, depending on which system you are using, some beta globulins migrate toward the cathode (Figure 1–4), reflecting the movement of the buffer toward the cathode. Depending on the amount of negative charge of the support medium, there will be an equal, relative, but opposite (positive) charge of the buffer adjacent to the support medium. This will pull the molecules that have a weaker negative charge, due to their lower isoelectric points, toward the cathode (Figure 1–4). It is important to realize that these molecules are not moving toward the cathode because they have a positive charge under the conditions of the assay; rather, they are just weak swimmers caught in a futile attempt to swim against the flow of a strong river.

Paper electrophoresis was slow, requiring several hours in order to achieve adequate separation of major protein fractions. Furthermore, it was opaque, gave poor resolution, and had significant problems with nonspecific protein adsorption [5]. Therefore, agar and cellulose acetate became popular stabilizing media for the clinical laboratories in the 1960s and 1970s. With these media, electrophoresis could be performed in less than an hour, and the clarity of the media facilitated densitometric scanning to estimate protein concentration.

Agar is a polysaccharide that is produced commercially by boiling red algae, filtering out the larger impurities, and removing the water-soluble impurities by freeze-thawing [6]. After precipitation in ethanol, the mixture con-

ENDOSMOTIC FLOW

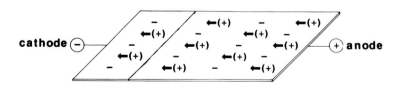

Figure 1–4. Endosmosis. Side view of electrophoresis illustrates negative charge of support medium and flow of positively charged buffer (+) to the cathode. Such flow affects migration of proteins in the support medium.

sists mainly of 1-4 linked 3,6-anhydro-alpha-L-galactose and 1-3 linked beta-D-galactose [7]. The final agar gel is a chemically complex structure, but for practical purposes it contains varying quantities of agarose and agaropectin. Agaropectin has a relatively high sulfate, pyruvate, and glucuronate content, which imparts a strong negative charge to the gel and results in considerable endosmotic flow, while agarose has few anionic groups [8].

Most commercial preparations of agar gels used for electrophoresis today contain relatively pure preparations of agarose. This minimizes both nonspecific adsorption of some proteins (such as beta lipoprotein and thyroglobulin) to the agar and the amount of endosmotic flow [9]. Although purified agarose preparations substantially reduce the endosmotic effect, it is probably fortunate that the preparations are still contaminated by a few negatively charged groups. Some endosmotic flow is desirable for electrophoresis of serum proteins, as it will conveniently pull the gamma globulins cathodally so the minor distortions present at the origin are irrelevant to interpretation of gamma region abnormalities.

For several years, cellulose acetate electrophoresis has been the most popular method for performing routine serum protein electrophoresis. The technique has several advantages over the earlier paper electrophoresis. As with agarose, only minimal adsorption of serum proteins occurs, and a sharper separation of the major serum protein bands is obtained much more quickly than by paper electrophoresis. However, it was recognized that the resolution on most cellulose acetate systems was inferior to that of agar gel electrophoresis [10]. This technique was popular in the clinical laboratory because of its simplicity, reproducibility, and reliable quantification of protein fractions by densitometry [11].

The successful replacement of paper electrophoresis by cellulose acetate electrophoresis was facilitated by the demonstration that accurate estimates could be made of each major protein fraction by simple densitometric scanning. In 1964, Briere and Mull [12] demonstrated that densitometric scanning of serum proteins separated by cellulose acetate electrophoresis gave the same measure of the major protein fractions as did elution and spectrophotometric measurement (Table 1-2).

Table 1-2   Comparison of Densitometric Scans on Cellulose Acetate with Eluted Protein Concentration

Method	Albumin	Alpha-1	Alpha-2	Beta	Gamma
Densitometry	4.5 ± 0.36	0.27 ± 0.08	0.62 ± 0.10	0.64 ± 0.12	0.95 ± 0.27
Elution	4.8 ± 0.34	0.22 ± 0.06	0.52 ± 0.09	0.59 ± 0.13	1.01 ± 0.25

Source: Data from Briere and Mull [12].
Note: Results expressed in g/100 ml.

Early Clinical Applications of Zone Electrophoresis

It was soon recognized that when tissues responsible for the synthesis or excretion of proteins were altered by disease, the resulting serum would produce distinctive electrophoretic patterns which could be helpful in diagnosis (Table 1-3). For instance, it was known as early as 1940 that in the nephrotic syndrome the serum contained markedly decreased levels of albumin and gamma globulin with increased levels of alpha-2 globulin [13]. At the same time, it was recognized that the urine from these patients contained the albumin lost from the serum as well as many other serum proteins. In reversible conditions such as minimal change nephropathy, then termed lipoid nephrosis, a return to the normal serum electrophoretic pattern was noted after resolution of the renal disease [14].

A small decrease in serum albumin was quickly recognized as a relatively nonspecific occurrence found in a variety of conditions that cause metabolic stress and as a feature of the acute phase reaction pattern (discussed later). However, the level of serum albumin in patients with liver disease gave clinically useful information because it was significantly correlated with the amount of tissue damage [15]. Further, it was noted that patients with severe liver disease had a broad elevation of gamma globulin [16], although the immunologic significance of that observation would not be understood for several years.

The single most important diagnosis one can make from serum protein electrophoresis is that of a monoclonal gammopathy. Today it is clear that a great heterogeneity of serum patterns can result from the neoplastic B-lympho-

Table 1-3 Early Clinical Use of Zone Electrophoresis

Clinical Diagnosis	Electrophoretic Pattern	Reference
Nephrotic syndrome	Decreased albumin, decreased gamma, increased alpha	Longsworth [13]
Liver disease	Decreased albumin, decreased beta,[a] increased gamma	Wajchenberg [15]
Myeloma	Increased gamma, decreased albumin	Reiner [18]
Agammaglobulinemia	Decreased gamma	Bruton [20]
Active systemic lupus erythematosus	Increased gamma	Coburn & Moore [22]
Multiple sclerosis, neurosyphilis	Increased CSF gamma	Kabat et al. [23]

[a]Decreased beta in massive liver necrosis.

cyte and plasma cell proliferations that occur in patients with chronic lymphocytic leukemia and multiple myeloma, respectively. Electrophoresis on the serum of patients with multiple myeloma could produce variable results. Most frequently, patients had elevated gamma globulin regions, although abnormalities could be seen anywhere from the alpha-1 through the gamma region. Also, the older zone electrophoresis techniques frequently could not detect any abnormality of serum proteins in these patients [17]. For instance, Reiner and Stern [18] found that 22% of patients with multiple myeloma that they studied had no significant abnormality in the serum. It was also soon recognized that many of these patients had Bence Jones proteins in their serum and, more frequently, in their urine. This could be detected by electrophoresis, although the amount of Bence Jones protein required for this detection was large by today's standards [19].

A major step forward in understanding the basic immunology of the human immune system involved the early application of serum protein electrophoresis by Colonel Ogden Bruton at the Walter Reed Army Medical Center [20]. One of his patients was a boy with a history of recurrent pyogenic infections. When protein electrophoresis was performed on this child's serum, it was discovered that the gamma globulin region was absent (actually, it was very low, but by the zone electrophoretic techniques available in 1952 it was undetectable). By using gamma globulin replacement therapy, Colonel Bruton was able to successfully treat this individual. Hence, although Colonel Bruton originally suspected that the disease was acquired rather than congenital (X-linked, as we now know), the disease correctly bears the name "Bruton's agammaglobulinemia." Early workers also recognized the existence of other forms of gamma globulin-related immunodeficiency that were correctly assumed to be acquired or that were congenital but transient. It was clear, for instance, that some infants who appeared to have Bruton's agammaglobulinemia recovered after 2-4 years; also, a profound hypogammaglobulinemia (today known as common variable immune deficiency) had surprisingly little clinical relevance for the young adults in whom it was detected [21].

Finally, Coburn and Moore [22] found that patients with clinically active systemic lupus erythematosus had elevated levels of gamma globulin. These findings preceded by 6 years the demonstration by Hargraves of the autoimmune phenomenon called the LE cell, and represent some of the earliest laboratory evidence suggesting the complicity of gamma globulin in the pathogenesis of this disease.

The availability of zone electrophoresis encouraged many investigators to examine a wide variety of fluids and extracts. Not surprisingly, urine was one of the first fluids studied. In patients with nephrotic syndrome, considerable albumin and some globulins could be seen at levels in the urine that gave a rough inverse correlation with the serum levels of these proteins [13]. Bence Jones proteins had long since been described by Dr. Henry Bence Jones, but with the advent of zone electrophoresis it became apparent that they had greater heterogeneity than previously thought. Although the Bence Jones proteins were always globulins, they migrated anywhere from the alpha through the gamma region. This finding raised important questions about the structure of these molecules, which were previously assumed to be homogeneous by virtue of their peculiar thermoprecipitating characteristics [19].

Because of the difficulty of diagnosing many central nervous system disorders, it was logical to use this new methodology to examine the cerebrospinal fluid. Analysis of concentrated cerebrospinal fluid from patients with multiple sclerosis and neurosyphilis showed markedly elevated gamma globulin content [23]. Similar elevations in the gamma globulin were found in central nervous system infections.

Despite these and many other observations, the clinical applications of zone electrophoresis were limited to obvious extreme elevations or reductions of major protein components. It was clear that many diseases were associated with more subtle alterations of proteins that were beyond the limitations of the early zone electrophoretic instruments. For protein electrophoresis to aid in the diagnosis of these conditions, better resolution of protein bands, simpler methods to quantify the fractions, and greater sensitivity were required.

With the earlier methods described previously, it was arguable whether agar gels could provide better resolution of the major protein bands than cellulose acetate. The heterogeneity of agar preparations and the ready availability of pure, commercially prepared cellulose acetate caused much wider usage of the latter. In addition, cellulose acetate allowed more rapid electrophoresis and could be dried, stained, and cleared more easily than agar [8].

Around 1970, however, reports appeared that described the advantages of the careful, high-resolution electrophoresis system described best by Wieme [9]. Many authors claimed that one could achieve diagnostically useful high resolution on agarose with techniques and equipment well within the capabilities of the clinical laboratory [24]. The availability of more highly purified agarose preparations, which minimized endosmotic flow and offered optical clarity and unimpeded migration due to their porosity, was credited with some of the improvement in resolution [25]. By the mid-1970s, using the modifications described in the next section, high-resolution agarose and cellulose acetate methodologies had evolved that facilitated the consistent demonstration of up to 12 distinct protein fractions.

At this point, I hope the discriminating reader is asking the critical managerial questions—"What is the clinical significance?" and "Is the test too costly?" These are key issues, not only because of the present environment of cost containment and reordered prospective payment plans, but because of standard principles of sound clinical judgment and laboratory medicine. Clinical tests should be based on well-documented criteria and used in specific decision-making processes. Unfortunately, all too often costly tests are requested and performed with only meager possibility of deriving useful information. Happily, the methods of high-resolution electrophoresis and immunofixation developed over the past decade have clearly answered these important medical and managerial concerns.

METHODS OF HIGH-RESOLUTION ELECTROPHORESIS

Principles of High-Resolution Electrophoresis

When proteins migrate in an electrical field, the extent of their migration and the degree of the resolution of each band depend on several factors. Some of the factors should be readily apparent from the discussion of protein structure. Two key factors in the migration of any protein are its pI and the pH of the buffer. The pI of any given protein is constant and dependent on its amino acid content. However, the charge that the protein expresses is determined by the pH of the solution in which it is dissolved. For instance, a protein such as fibrinogen has a pI of 5.5. In an electrophoresis buffer with a pH of 8.6, it donates protons to the buffer and is left with a net negative charge.

When we want to look at the features of high-resolution electrophoresis (HRE), we are concerned with the ability to discriminate between separate but closely migrating major protein components. Now we must consider several other important factors inherent in the particular electrophoresis system that we adopt. These factors include velocity of migration, passive diffusion, and interactions of proteins with the supporting medium. Each can be influenced by adjusting the variables in the electrophoretic system. Excellent detailed discussions of these factors are available in Wieme and Bier [9, 12].

The speed with which a protein migrates in an electric field (electrophoretic mobility) under defined conditions of pH, ionic strength, temperature, and voltage is characteristic for that protein. The formula defining the variables involved in calculating the electrophoretic mobility (μ) of a protein is

$$\mu = \frac{d}{Et}$$

where d is the distance traveled from the origin in centimeters, E is the strength of the electrical field in V/cm, and t is the period of electrophoresis in seconds. As the strength of the electrical field is inversely proportional to its length, that is, V/cm, a shorter support medium will permit faster separation of proteins.

Although stronger voltage will give a faster separation of proteins, unfortunately it also results in more heat generation, which is deleterious to resolution of individual bands. The amount of heat generated (in joules) when the electric current passes through the apparatus can be calculated by:

$$\text{Heat generated} = \frac{xE^2}{A}$$

where x is the specific conductance of the apparatus, E is the strength of the electric field in V/cm, and A is the mechanical heat equivalent. From this it is clear that heat production increases exponentially as the voltage is increased.

This excessive heat production plays havoc with good resolution of electrophoretic bands. One of the major effects of heat is to increase the thermal agitation and hence the diffusion of the protein molecules. Diffusion has the effect of broadening the width of a band and thereby decreasing the resolution. Heat production can also decrease the viscosity of the medium. Although this does permit a more rapid electrophoretic migration (μ) of the proteins through the gel, it is more than counterbalanced by an even greater increase in diffusion with a resulting decrease in resolution. Before closed systems were common, the heat generated further complicated resolution by causing enough evaporation to change ionic strength.

The ionic strength of the buffer is also an important factor in the resolution of individual protein bands. As the concentration of the salt ions in a buffer increases, the velocity of electrophoretic migration decreases for each protein being assayed. There is no effect, however, on the relative migration of serum proteins as the result of ionic strength. The effect of ionic concentration on the migration of proteins in the electric field is largely the result of interaction of the buffer ions with the surface charges on the protein.

Consider a buffer in which we increase the concentration of NaCl. At the typical pH 8.6 of agar gel electrophoresis, human serum albumin has a negative surface charge. The positive sodium ions are attracted to the negative charges on the albumin and diminish its effective net negative charge in the solution. Further, positively charged ions now in immediate proximity to the albumin are attracted toward the cathode during electrophoresis and tend to retard the progress of albumin toward the anode. This accumulation of positive charges in the buffer around the negatively charged albumin is known as the diffuse double layer. This is why it is important to control evaporation with resultant concentration of ions in the buffer during electrophoresis [9].

Another factor limiting the effective separation of protein bands is adsorption of the molecules to the agar gel itself. Because of the negative charges possessed by the relatively purified agarose solutions used today, pH < 5.0 are impracticable. Below this pH, serum proteins would have a positive charge and would precipitate in the gel.

With better control of such details as buffer strength, voltage, heat dissipation, purity of the agarose or cellulose acetate, and gel thickness, the HRE systems we describe provide 12 distinct protein bands, which encompass more than 95% of serum proteins [26]. These methods are better able to delineate clinically significant deficiencies of serum proteins such as alpha-1 antitrypsin, and are considerably more sensitive for detecting monoclonal gammopathies than the five-band separation previously used in clinical laboratories [27].

High-Resolution Electrophoresis on Agarose

To achieve high resolution, the method of Wieme as modified by Johansson [5] is commonly used with agarose. A 1% concentration of agarose is used in

0.075 *M*, pH 8.6 barbital buffer containing 2 m*M* calcium lactate. Commercially available agarose slides have a uniform thin (1 mm) layer of agarose on an inert plastic support (Grafar, Panagel, Helena, Beckman, Corning, and others).

The application of the sample to the gel is critically important to achieving proper separation and reproducible results. The specimen must be applied to the agarose surface in a very narrow band. First, excess moisture is removed from the surface of the gel by blotting with filter paper. A plastic mask with uniform 1 × 14 mm slits for sample application is firmly layered onto the blotted gel. It is important that the mask be rinsed with distilled water and evenly applied to the surface of the agarose so that no air pockets are present; these may distort the application of the sample. With such a narrow application, even minor distortions will result in preparations that are difficult or impossible to interpret (Figure 1-5). Five microliters of sample are placed over each slit and allowed to diffuse into the gel for 7 minutes. Attention to detail in sample application is important as the final band width and configuration are determined by the initial application.

After sample application is complete, the gels are placed so that their plastic backing is in direct contact with a cooling block (typically kept at 4°C prior to electrophoresis). The cooling block must be properly prepared and stored; if it is not at the proper temperature, the heat generated from the high voltages applied to these samples will produce the effects described above and poor resolution of bands will result. In some systems, it is possible to have too much buffer in the reservoir. In these cases, when the migrating gamma region reaches the buffer, it will form an artifactual slow gamma band (Figure 1-6).

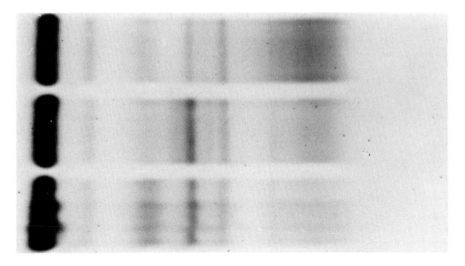

Figure 1-5. High-resolution electrophoretic strip of three serum samples stained with Amido black. Note distortion in bands of third sample. The occurrence of the distortion in all bands indicates that this is an artifact due to an application problem.

Most high-resolution electrophoresis (HRE) systems in agarose run with an electrical field of about 20 V/cm (a setting of 200 V for each 10-cm length of agarose) and a current of about 100–120 mA. Under these conditions, the typical run lasts 30–50 minutes.

When electrophoresis has been completed, the agarose sheet is placed into an acetic acid-picric acid solution to fix the proteins. The fixative solution is made by dissolving 1.5 g of picric acid in 120 ml of 17% aqueous acetic acid. (The reader should note that picric acid is a hazardous substance that can become highly explosive when stored for long periods of time [28]. Good

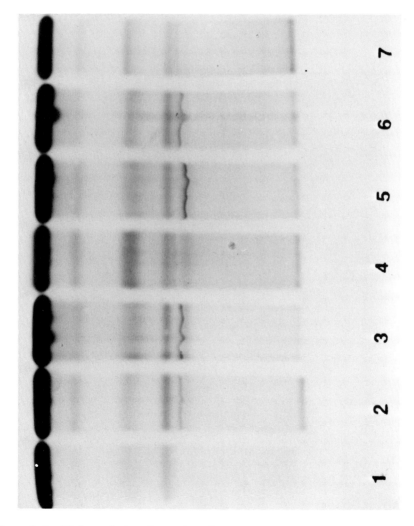

Figure 1–6. High-resolution electrophoretic strip with eight samples stained with crystal violet. All samples appear to have a small, slow gamma restriction, which may be mistaken for a monoclonal band. This artifact results from excess buffer in the reservoir.

laboratory technique including checking bottle dates and crystallization around bottle caps will minimize the danger.)

After fixing the proteins for 10 minutes, the gel is given two 3-minute rinses in 5% acetic acid. A sharkskin filter paper moistened with 5% acetic acid is placed over the surface of the gel followed by three or four blotters. A 1-kg flat weight is used to press the gel to facilitate rapid, even drying. The gel is then dried with a gentle stream of hot air for 5–10 minutes.

For examination of serum and urine proteins, we prefer staining the gel with Amido black. While both Coomassie brilliant blue and Amido black give distinct patterns, the Amido black has less background between major bands, which makes interpretation of serum and urine electrophoretic patterns more straightforward [5]. Part of the difference is that Coomassie brilliant blue is more sensitive than Amido black and stains small protein molecules at these sites. For cerebrospinal fluid, where sensitivity can be a problem even after concentrating a sample 80-fold, we use Coomassie brilliant blue. With Amido black staining, the gel is placed in a 0.1% solution of Amido black in 5% acetic acid for 10 minutes, followed by destaining with a solution of 10% glacial acetic acid, 30% methanol, and 60% distilled water for 1, 10, and 10 minutes, respectively. The gel is dried and examined both directly and by densitometry.

High-Resolution Electrophoresis on Cellulosic Media

In the past 5 years, newer preparations of cellulose acetate membranes and staining techniques have allowed the clinical laboratory to perform HRE on cellulose acetate membranes. It is still controversial whether the resolution on this system is equivalent to that seen with the agarose systems; however, the technique can separate serum proteins into 10 or 12 fractions that are useful in clinical diagnosis [29–31]. Furthermore, the same technique can be used for immunofixation analysis as with the agarose method.

Densitometric Scanning of High-Resolution Electrophoresis

There is unanimity that HRE gels should be evaluated by direct visual inspection after staining. No group advocates solely performing densitometric scanning with interpretation merely from the scan and percentages generated. Some groups even recommend that densitometric study not be performed [31]. This reflects recognition of important yet subtle changes that can more easily be discerned with direct visual examination of the stained electrophoretic strip by an experienced observer than by a densitometric scan. For instance, in the case shown in Figure 1–7, a small but distinct area of restricted mobility is present in the slow gamma area of sample X. However, the densitometric scan from this sample (Figure 1–8) shows only a minimal distortion, which may be

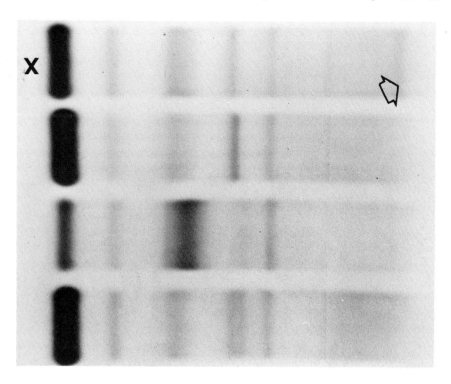

Figure 1–7. Top sample (X) has a small but obvious slow gamma restriction (*arrow*) that occurs in none of the other samples. This type of restriction is usually a small monoclonal protein.

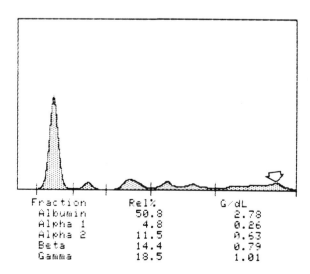

Fraction	Rel%	G/dL
Albumin	50.8	2.78
Alpha 1	4.8	0.26
Alpha 2	11.5	0.63
Beta	14.4	0.79
Gamma	18.5	1.01

Figure 1–8. Densitometric scan of top sample from Figure 1–7. The slow gamma region shows a subtle restriction (*arrow*).

missed; this turned out to be a monoclonal IgG kappa protein. Therefore, the electrophoretic strip should always be examined directly.

Densitometric scanning of serum protein electrophoretic patterns has been useful in providing quantitative information about the major protein fractions. It has been widely accepted by clinicians and already allows for utilization of a microcomputer in interpretation or scanning the sample [32–34]. Furthermore, all groups that suggested direct visual examination of the stained strip as preferable to densitometric scanning emphasized that the strip must be examined by an experienced observer. Unfortunately, there is no uniform agreement on what criteria determine an experienced observer.

Many laboratories are not so fortunate to have such experienced observers and most have no more than one or two. One can expect that there is going to be some day-to-day variation, especially when more than one individual interpret the electrophoretic strips. Therefore, we believe that densitometry is a useful *adjunct* in interpreting HRE patterns. For example, the HRE strip from a recent run is shown in Figure 1–9. The observer originally called sample Y normal when he just looked at the strip. However, the densitometric scan (Figure 1–10) indicated that there was a significantly decreased percentage of protein in the alpha-1 fraction. This caused reexamination of the strip and further studies that documented that the patient had an abnormal alpha-1 antitrypsin phenotype.

Densitometry is helpful in the interpretation of HRE patterns for making patient care decisions. It has its limitations, and, therefore, a straightforward commonsense approach is helpful. The approach we advocate is to examine each case by *both* direct visual examination of the stained strip and densitometric scanning. We examine the strips first visually and then use the densitometric scan to confirm our impressions when an increase or decrease in a

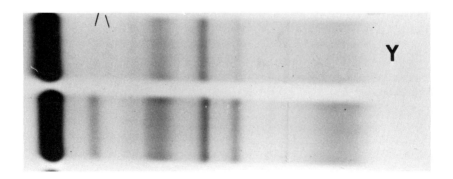

Figure 1–9. High-resolution electrophoresis (HRE) of two serum samples. Sample Y has an abnormal alpha-1 region. Instead of the prominent single band seen in the lower serum, sample Y has two faint bands (*lines*).

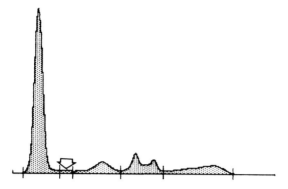

Figure 1-10.   Densitometric scan of sample Y from Figure 1-9. The low alpha-1 region (*arrow*) helped alert the interpreter to the deficiency. Alpha-1 region deficiency is best detected by direct examination of the strip, but useful adjunctive information obtained from densitometry helps to prevent errors.

region is marginal. When following patients with a monoclonal gammopathy, the densitometric scan provides us with excellent quantitative information in most cases [35]. Obvious exceptions are migration of the monoclonal protein near other prominent bands such as C3 or transferrin.

Also, it is important to recognize the limitations of the technique. When one scans the alpha-1 globulin region, or any region with only 5% or less of the total serum protein, changes of the baseline or distortion of the gel pattern can give erroneous results. For instance, if the alpha-1 region appeared low on direct visual inspection of the electrophoretic strip and the densitometric scan recorded that the "measured" value of the alpha-1 region was in the low-normal range, one should still recommend further studies to exclude the possibility of alpha-1 antitrypsin deficiency. This recognizes the inherent inaccuracy when measuring in the low range. With this, as in the case demonstrated in Figures 1-9 and 1-10, quantitative information can be helpful.

We perform densitometric scanning on all serum HRE patterns. In our laboratory, we dilute the serum sample 1:4 in the electrophoresis buffer to prevent overloading of the agarose gel. After it is stained with Amido black as previously described, the gel is dried and scanned. When performing scans on the Gelman ACD-18 densitometer, the scan length is 65–75 mm with the OD range set at 2. Gels are scanned by a 575-nm wavelength through a slit dimension of 0.2 × 3.0 mm. When using the Beckman Appraise, the scan length is 66 mm with the 600 filter; gain is set at 125 and the track spacing is 13 mm. Despite the fact that HRE allows visualization of 12 bands, we chose to use a standard five-serum-fraction pattern. This reflected the considerable variation in small bands such as beta-1 lipoprotein and alpha-1 antichymotrypsin. A comparison with our former routine five-band cellulose acetate

Table 1-4 Comparison of Normal Serum Protein Values by Cellulose Acetate versus High-Resolution Electrophoresis Densitometry

Serum Fraction	Cellulose Acetate	High Resolution
Albumin	3.54–5.0[a]	4.11–5.39[b]
Alpha-1	0.21–0.34	0.10–0.24
Alpha-2	0.40–0.75	0.33–0.73
Beta[c]	0.73–1.07	0.57–1.05
Gamma	0.66–1.32	0.62–1.33

[a]Results expressed as 2 SD.
[b]Beckman Appraise Densitometer used for scanning.
[c]Although the high-resolution scans can be separated into two beta fractions, only one is used for comparison with the five-band pattern.

technique disclosed a lower level of alpha-1 and alpha-2 globulins in the Amido black-stained HRE strips compared to the Ponceau S-stained cellulose acetate (Table 1-4). However, the superior band discrimination by the Amido black stain made this difference in densitometric information insignificant for the purpose of clinical interpretation.

It is clear from earlier studies that densitometric scans of Amido black-stained electrophoresis strips provided a linear estimate of human serum albumin, transferrin, and gamma globulin [36]. Although most workers found a relatively decreased uptake of this dye by gamma globulin as compared to other fractions, this does not interfere with deriving quantitative estimates of gamma globulins from the densitometric scans. For example, we determined that there is excellent agreement between the densitometric scans and nephelometric measurements of IgG using the serum of patients having gamma-migrating IgG monoclonal gammopathies. Therefore, the densitometric scan is used to follow these patients (Figure 1-11). Since most of the monoclonal lesions secrete proteins that migrate in the gamma region, this provides a convenient method for follow-up of these patients. However, when the monoclonal protein migrates in the alpha- or beta-globulin regions, densitometry is not as useful. The other major proteins such as haptoglobin, alpha-2 macroglobulin, transferrin, and C3 that are found in these regions interfere with this method. In Chapter 2, more specific aspects of diagnosis using both direct visualization of the electrophoretic strips and information derived from the densitometric scans are presented.

HIGH-RESOLUTION ELECTROPHORESIS VERSUS STANDARD ELECTROPHORESIS

Routine five-band serum protein electrophoretic patterns have been and will continue to be useful for many years. In deciding whether or not to adopt an HRE method in a clinical laboratory setting, one must be concerned with the

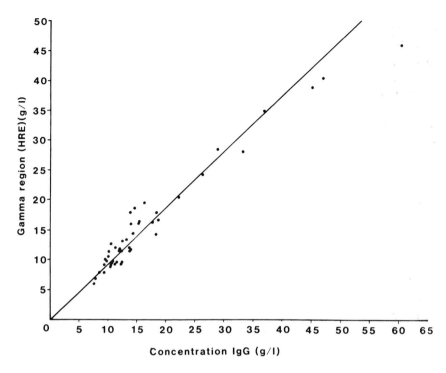

Figure 1-11. Correlation of gamma region concentration, as determined by densitometric scans of HRE gels, with total IgG as determined by nephelometry. Samples were serum from patients with known gamma-migrating monoclonal gammopathies. The excellent correlation demonstrates why we follow these patients with HRE and densitometric scans only rather than repeating immunoglobulin quantification and/or immunofixation.

potential for diagnoses not previously possible. Are the conditions now detectable relevant to the patients seen in your practice? What is the cost of the procedure? Are the technical requirements so strict as to make reproducibility in a clinical laboratory setting impractical?

Of the many important conditions that one can diagnose by examining the serum protein electrophoresis patterns, the most dramatic and clinically significant is the diagnosis of a monoclonal gammopathy. This demonstration means that the patient has a neoplastic proliferation of plasma cells. The amount of the monoclonal protein together with clinical evaluation of the patient's bone marrow, blood, and radiologic studies will help the clinician decide whether the patient has multiple myeloma, monoclonal gammopathy of undetermined significance, Waldenstrom's macroglobulinemia, or another B-cell proliferative disease. Yet, the literature notes that as many as 15–20% of patients with myeloma had normal serum protein electrophoresis patterns when examined by the standard five-band technique [37]. Although some of these cases may reflect the rare nonsecretory myeloma, or the more common light chain disease with most of the monoclonal protein passing into the urine (usually creating a hypogammaglobulinemia most easily detectable by high-resolution techniques; see Chapter 2), many cases reflect the inherent insensitivity of the method.

With HRE techniques, detection of monoclonal gammopathies has become manyfold more sensitive than it was with five-band electrophoresis methods. Small monoclonal proteins that were entirely undetected by earlier methods can be detected by this technique. While many of these smaller monoclonal bands fall into the category of "monoclonal gammopathy of undetermined significance," they are clearly *not* all benign monoclonal gammopathies. Some represent early multiple myeloma; others represent monoclonal proteins that are seen in association with common B-cell neoplasms such as chronic lymphocytic leukemia or well-differentiated lymphocytic lymphoma (see Chapter 5). Still others have been associated with autoimmune disease and peripheral neuropathies.

With the present techniques, when the densitometric scan of the gamma globulin region is below normal in an adult suspected of having a lymphoproliferative disease, the interpreter can make important suggestions for further testing such as looking for Bence Jones proteins in the urine or performing immunofixation to look for small monoclonal proteins associated with B-lymphocyte neoplasms. With the greater sensitivity of these techniques one can detect a relapse of myeloma in patients being followed for response to chemotherapy.

Beyond the importance of the present techniques with neoplastic conditions, one can more easily detect other clinically important serum protein abnormalities. With the five-band electrophoretic methods, the alpha-1 lipoprotein, alpha-1 antitrypsin, and genetic variants of alpha-1 antitrypsin all spread diffusely in the alpha-1 region. Now one can detect a decrease in the specific alpha-1 antitrypsin band even in the presence of an increased level of alpha-1 lipoprotein, which formerly masked detection of this important enzyme deficiency (Chapter 2). Also, one can detect genetic variants of this enzyme inhibitor, which may give important information for kindreds of the patient.

Classical patterns of liver disease, renal disease, and acute phase reaction are much clearer with HRE than by previous methodology. HRE also allows detection of oligoclonal bands in the cerebrospinal fluid of patients with multiple sclerosis and thereby provides the clinician with the single most reliable confirmatory test of this condition (Chapter 3). In examining urine specimens, an HRE study will discriminate between tubular and glomerular damage in a patient with proteinuria. These and many other applications discussed in detail later in this volume demonstrate the clinical relevance of this method.

But what about the cost? Today the clinical laboratory is being asked not just to use the most modern methods of diagnosis, but to justify the cost for newer equipment, additional reagents, and the high level of training required for the proper use of this sophisticated apparatus. Rightly so! If the physician wants to try a new, unproven procedure that has marginal worth, he or she should pay for it. Although many of the new reimbursement guidelines are difficult, we laboratorians cannot be so naive as to think that they are totally unwarranted. It is time for the laboratorian to help in cost containment by using the expertise it has taken us so long to acquire.

How does HRE help in cost containment? The gels themselves cost more than most of the available gels for the older five-band patterns, while the technical expertise to perform either assay and the stains cost about the same. The savings derive from two major factors. First, the sensitivity of the technique allows the interpreter to detect conditions that would have been missed by less sensitive methods. Findings such as alpha-1 antitrypsin deficiency, oligoclonal gamma bands in multiple sclerosis, small monoclonal bands in patients with B-lymphocyte neoplasms and peripheral neuropathies, and proteinuria patterns could not be distinguished with older methods. Detecting these and other abnormalities (see Chapters 2–5) can have considerable importance in streamlining the workup of the patient. Second, the sensitivity of the high-resolution electrophoresis technique together with immunoglobulin quantification procedures available today allow the interpreter to determine the presence or absence of a monoclonal gammopathy without performing more expensive, time-consuming procedures such as serum immunoelectrophoresis. In our institution, we have eliminated over two-thirds of the speciality procedures such as immunoelectrophoresis or immunofixation performed on serum. Our strategy for streamlining these procedures is detailed in Chapter 5.

It is difficult to calculate the savings achieved by such efficiencies. However, recent publications have looked more carefully into the role of identifying "true" costs of medical care. Conn et al. [38] noted that the Laboratory Workload Recording Method from the College of American Pathologists offers a way both to calculate the costs of performing particular procedures and to project the costs of alternative management action. Others have pointed out the importance of reviewing the efficiency of laboratory utilization to prevent overordering [39]. The use of HRE has increased the cost of electrophoretic procedures less than 10% while providing the basis for accelerating the diagnostic process for patients with myeloma and other lymphoproliferative disease by 2 days for most and as much as a week for some. It has allowed us to eliminate redundant, expensive immunoelectrophoresis and immunofixation in many cases (both inpatient and outpatient). Finally, its sensitivity has allowed us to detect more accurately a wide variety of serum protein abnormalities.

The expanded use of this technique will be important both in decreasing unnecessary, expensive testing in the laboratory and in using the expertise of the laboratorian with interpretive reporting to facilitate diagnoses. Therefore, let us consider the practical diagnostic applications of HRE and immunofixation, which can diagnose conditions earlier (at more treatable stages), more quickly (a 1-day procedure rather than one requiring 3 or more days, thereby reducing hospital costs), and more accurately compared to our previous methodology.

REFERENCES

1. Tiselius A. A new apparatus for electrophoretic analysis of colloidal mixtures. Trans Faraday Soc 1932;33:524–531.
2. Tiselius A. Introduction. In: Bier M, ed. Electrophoresis, theory, methods and applications. New York: Academic Press, 1959:xv–xix.
3. Kunkel HG, Tiselius A. Electrophoresis of proteins on filter paper. J Gen Physiol 1951;35:89–118.
4. McDonald HJ, Spitzer RH. Polyvinylpyrrolidine: the electromigration characteristics of the blood plasma expander. Circ Res 1953;1:396–404.
5. Johansson BG. Agarose gel electrophoresis. Scand J Clin Lab Invest 1972;29 [Suppl]124:7–21.
6. Serwer P. Agarose gels: properties and use for electrophoresis. Electrophoresis 1983;4:375–382.
7. Rees DA. Structure, conformation, and mechanism in the formation of polysaccharide gels and networks. In: Wolfrom ML, Tipson RS, Horton D, eds. Advances in carbohydrate chemistry and biochemistry. New York: Academic Press, 1969;24:267–332.
8. Nerenberg ST. Electrophoretic screening procedures. Philadelphia: Lea and Febiger, 1973.
9. Wieme RJ. Agar gel electrophoresis. Amsterdam: Elsevier, 1965.
10. Cawley LP, Minard B, Penn GM. Electrophoresis and immunochemical reactions in gels. Techniques and interpretations. Chicago:ASCP Press, 1978.
11. Kohn J. Small-scale membrane filter electrophoresis and immunoelectrophoresis. Clin Chim Acta 1958;3:450–454.
12. Briere RO, Mull JD. Electrophoresis of serum protein with cellulose acetate. A method for quantitation. Am J Clin Pathol 1964;34:547–551.
13. Longsworth LG, MacInnes DA. Electrophoretic study of nephrotic sera and urine. J Exp Med 1940;71:77–86.
14. Lenke SE, Berger HM. Abrupt improvement of serum electrophoretic pattern in nephrosis after ACTH-induced diuresis. Proc Soc Exp Biol Med 1951;78:366–369.
15. Wajhenberg BL, Hoxter G, Segal J, Mattar E, de Ulhoa Cintra AB, Montenegro MR, Pontes JF. Electrophoretic patterns of the plasma proteins in diffuse liver necrosis. Gastroenterology 1956;30:882–893.
16. Franklin M, Bean WB, Paul WD, Routh JI, de la Hueraga J, Popper H. Electrophoretic studies in liver disease. I. Comparison of serum and plasma electrophoretic patterns in liver disease, with special reference to fibrinogen and gamma globulin patterns. J Clin Invest 1951;30:718–728.
17. Moore DH. Clinical and physiological applications of electrophoresis. In: Bier M, ed. Electrophoresis theory, methods and applications. New York: Academic Press, 1959:369–425.
18. Reiner M, Stern KG. Electrophoretic studies on the protein distribution in the serum of multiple myeloma patients. Acta Haematol (Basel) 1953;9:19–29.
19. Moore DJ. Kabat EA, Gutman AB. Bence-Jones proteinemia in multiple myeloma. J Clin Invest 1943;22:67–75.

20. Bruton OC. Agammaglobulinemia. Pediatrics 1952;9:722–727.
21. Gitlin D. Low resistance to infection: relationship to abnormalities in gamma globulins. Bull NY Acad Med 1955;31:359–365.
22. Coburn AF, Moore DH. The plasma proteins in disseminated lupus erythematosus. Bull Johns Hopkins Hosp 1943;73:196–214.
23. Kabat EA, Moore DH, Landow H. An electrophoretic study of the protein components in cerebrospinal fluid and their relationship to the serum proteins. J Clin Invest 1942;21:571–577.
24. Rosenfeld L. Serum protein electrophoresis: a comparison of the use of thin-layer agarose gel and cellulose acetate. Am J Clin Pathol 1974;62:702–706.
25. Elevitch FR, Aronson SB, Feichtmeir TV, Enterline ML. Thin gel electrophoresis in agarose. Am J Clin Pathol 1966;46:692–697.
26. Laurell CB. Electrophoresis, specific protein assays or both in measurement of plasma proteins. Clin Chem 1973;19:99–102.
27. Howanitz PJ. Monoclonal protein detection: a comparison of two electrophoretic methods. Clin Chem 1977;23:1137 (Abstr).
28. Safety note. Clin Chem 1980;26:804.
29. Ojala K, Weber TH. Some alternatives to the proposed selected method for "agarose gel electrophoresis." Clin Chem 1980; 26:1754–1755.
30. Janik B, Dane RG. High resolution electrophoresis of serum proteins on cellulosic membranes and identification of individual components by immunofixation and immunosubtraction. J Clin Chem Clin Biochem 1981;19:712–713.
31. Aguzzi F, Jayakar AD, Merlini G, Petrini C. Electrophoresis: cellulose acetate vs. agarose gel, visual inspection vs. densitometry. Clin Chem 1981;27:1944–1945.
32. Knuppel VW, Neumeier D, Fateh-Moghadam A, Knedel M. Rechnerunterstutzte befundung von eiwei Belekrophoresen auf celluloseacetatfolie. J Clin Chem Clin Biochem 1984;22:407–417.
33. Talamo ST, Losos FJ, Kessler GF. Microcomputer-assisted interpretative reporting of protein electrophoresis data. Am J Clin Pathol 1982;77:726–730.
34. Tracy RP, Young DS. A densitometer based on a microcomputer and TV camera for use in the clinical laboratory. Clin Chem 1984;30:462–465.
35. Keren DF, Di Sante AC, Bordine SL. Densitometric scanning of high resolution electrophoresis of serum: methodology and clinical application. Am J Clin Pathol 1986;85:348–352.
36. Uriel J. Interpretation quantitative des resultats spres electrophorese en gelose, I. Considerations generales, application a l'etude de constituants proteiques isoles. Clin Chem Acta 1958;3:234–238.
37. Kyle RA. Multiple myeloma review of 869 cases. Mayo Clin Proc 1974;50:29–40.
38. Conn RB, Aller RD, Lundberg GD. Identifying costs of medical care. An essential step in allocating resources. JAMA 1985;253:1586–1589.
39. McConnell TS, Berger PR, Dayton HH, Umland BE, Skipper BE. Professional review of laboratory utilization. Hum Pathol 1982;13:399–403.

CHAPTER 2

Serum Proteins Identified by High-Resolution Electrophoresis

The electrophoretic patterns produced from high-resolution electrophoresis (HRE) allow the laboratorian to make a more sophisticated appraisal of several clinically relevent conditions than was possible with earlier electrophoretic techniques. Unfortunately, the greater number of bands that are present with HRE can be intimidating until one becomes familiar with the most common patterns and genetic variants which occur. Fear not! Many proteins visualized are already familiar to observers of older electrophoretic techniques. The more subtle bands that can be recognized on HRE are discussed in this chapter with pertinent case examples in Chapter 6.

While the older five-band electrophoretic patterns are useful in diagnosing extreme pathologic states such as advanced cirrhosis, nephrotic syndrome, and myeloma, the newer HRE methods have vastly expanded the diagnostic capability of the clinical laboratory. With HRE, one can detect small minimonoclonal proteins in patients with B-cell neoplasms, oligoclonal bands in the cerebrospinal fluid of patients with multiple sclerosis, circulating immune complexes, alpha-1 antitrypsin deficiencies, glomerular and tubular proteinuria patterns, and several genetic and drug-related abnormalities.

Clearly, some protein abnormalities give more clinically useful information than do others. In this chapter, we delineate the protein bands that can be seen in serum using this technique and the usual circumstances of their increase, decrease, or change in mobility or band architecture. Relevant band patterns seen in disease states are then reviewed in Chapter 3. By optimal application of the HRE technique, the clinical laboratory can spare patients needless expense such as that of immunoelectrophoresis or immunofixation when it is not required. Further, by skillfully interpreting the information obtained, the laboratorian can speed up the relevant diagnostic process.

PROTEINS IDENTIFIED BY HIGH-RESOLUTION ELECTROPHORESIS

The protein bands identified by high-resolution electrophoresis (HRE) of serum are, for convenience, arbitrarily divided into major and minor protein bands (Tables 2–1 and 2–2). In our system, the major bands constitute those which are virtually always seen in normal serum. Minor bands are those that are very weak in normal serum and/or affect the electrophoretic pattern in a variety of disease states or genetic variants. The exact position of some of the bands will vary slightly with the methodology employed, and separation of some bands such as alpha-2 macroglobulin from haptoglobin is incomplete with HRE.

Prealbumin

Prealbumin is the first band encountered on the anodal side of the electrophoresis strip. It has a molecular weight of 55,000 and is known to function in transporting thyroxine. With most HRE procedures, this protein produces only a weak, diffuse band just proximal to albumin (Figure 2–1). It may have other physiologic functions and has been shown to play a role in familial amyloidosis [1].

With a serum concentration of 10–40 mg/dl and the typical 1:2 or 1:4 dilution of serum, prealbumin is beneath the level where its increase or decrease can be analyzed by serum protein electrophoresis. However, prealbumin is a more substantial fraction of cerebrospinal fluid and is considered further in Chapter 3.

Table 2–1   Major Protein Bands

Protein	Concentration[a]	Function
Albumin	4.0–5.0	Transport/oncotic
Alpha-1 antitrypsin	100–400	Protease inhibitor
Haptoglobin	20–200	Binds hemoglobin
Alpha-2 macroglobulin	175–400	Protease inhibitor
Transferrin	200–400	Binds iron
C3	80–250	Host defense
Fibrinogen	300–500[b]	Thrombosis
Immunoglobulins		Host defense
IgA —beta	25–390	
IgM—origin	20–390	
IgG —gamma	600–1600	

[a]Concentration in gm/dl for albumin and in mg/dl for all other proteins.
[b]Concentration in plasma.

Table 2–2 Minor Protein Bands

Proteins	Concentration[a]	Function
Prealbumin	10–40	Transport
Alpha-1 lipoprotein –[b]	250–400	High-density lipoproteins
Alpha-1 acid glycoprotein	50–150	Acute phase
Inter-alpha-trypsin inhibitor	20–70	Protease inhibitor
Group-specific component	20–50	Carrier protein
Pregnancy zone protein	0.5–2.0	Increase in pregnancy
Alpha-1 antichymotrypsin	30–60	Protease inhibitor
Ceruloplasmin	15–60	Copper binding
Fibronectin	15–30	Wound healing
Beta lipoprotein	200–700	Low-density lipoprotein
C4	20–60	Host defense
C-reactive protein	<2	Inflammation

[a]Concentration in mg/dl.
[b]Difficult to see in normal samples due to diffuse migration.

Albumin

Albumin is the most prominent protein in the normal serum protein electrophoresis. Roughly reflecting its prominence in serum, albumin serves important functions such as accounting for much of the osmotic effect of plasma

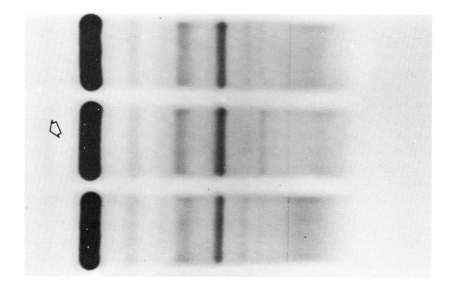

Figure 2–1. Prealbumin can be seen as a faint band (*arrow*) just anodal to albumin. By this technique, the prealbumin is too indistinct to judge its increase or decrease.

proteins. Albumin transports a variety of endogenous and exogenous molecules such as bilirubin, enzymes, hormones, lipid, metallic ions, and drugs. Many of these would be poorly soluble in aqueous solution alone. The breadth of the normal albumin band is due to both the great serum concentration and its microheterogeneity which results from the charges and size of various molecules being transported by albumin [2]. The marked tendency for albumin to transport a variety of substances accounts for some of the abnormal patterns of electrophoresis in patients receiving albumin-binding drugs or those with hyperbilirubinemia (Figure 2–2).

Decreased Albumin

Decreased concentration of serum albumin indicates significant pathology either in the production of albumin by the liver or its leakage through a damaged surface: glomerular disease, gastrointestinal loss, or thermal injury (Table 2–3). In western countries, a decrease in the production of albumin most commonly reflects severe liver injury. Because of the large reserve capacity of the liver, hypoalbuminemia resulting from liver damage occurs after most of the hepatocytes have been damaged or destroyed. Such a decrease is usually

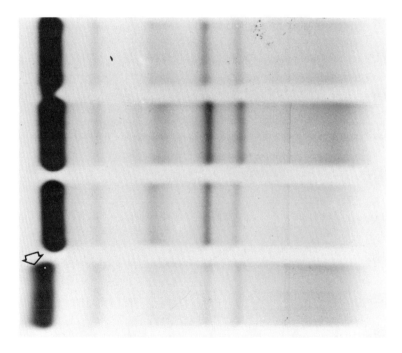

Figure 2–2.   Bottom electrophoretic sample is from patient with hyperbilirubinemia. Bilirubin binds to the albumin, resulting in anodal slurring (*arrow*).

Table 2-3 Alterations of Serum Albumin

Alteration	*Pathophysiology*
Analbuminemia	Congenital
Bisalbuminemia	Congenital
Hypoalbuminemia	A. Decreased production
	1. Liver disease
	2. Protein malnutrition
	3. Acute inflammation
	B. Increased loss
	1. Kidney disease
	2. Protein-losing enteropathy
	3. Thermal injury
Anodal smearing	Binding with anionic molecules
	1. Bilirubin
	2. Heparin
	3. Penicillin, etc.

accompanied by clotting abnormalities and decreased synthesis of other hepatocyte products including alpha-1 antitrypsin, haptoglobin, and transferrin (Figure 2-2) [3]. In Third World countries, severe protein malnutrition (kwashiorkor) is the leading cause of decreased synthesis of albumin. Patients with neoplasia or other chronic diseases also develop a nutritionally related hypoalbuminemia.

Analbuminemia, decreased or absent synthesis of albumin due to inheritance of recessive genes, is extremely rare. Surprisingly, the few patients with analbuminemia who have been reported are clinically well, presumably due to the maintenance of oncotic pressure and transport function by other serum proteins [4,5]. However, some patients have mild edema that is controlled with diuretics [6]. Another rare inherited abnormality of albumin is bisalbuminemia in which two types of albumin that have slightly different electrophoretic mobility are produced; this results in two distinct and usually equal peaks in the albumin region. These patients are clinically well.

A decreased concentration of serum albumin also results from excessive loss through injury to the kidneys, gastrointestinal tract, thermal injury to the skin, or severe eczema, and in hypercatabolic states. When renal damage is severe enough to allow albumin to pass in large amounts into the urine, there is a corresponding loss of other serum proteins, including gamma globulins, into the urine [7]. Some of the largest serum proteins, such as alpha-2 macroglobulin with a molecular weight of 1,000,000, remain in the serum and are synthesized at an increased rate. The latter constitutes the body's attempt to stabilize oncotic pressure.

Gastrointestinal loss in various protein-losing enteropathies is also associated with hypoalbuminemia and a decrease in concentration of other serum proteins. As with the nephrotic pattern, alpha-2 globulin typically is normal or elevated [8]. Absolute distinction between gastrointestinal loss of protein and renal loss cannot be made by examining the electrophoretic strips; this is one example of a situation in which clinical information is needed to optimize the interpretation of the patterns seen. We are trained in pattern recognition for disease states and many genetic variants; we are not soothsayers. When in doubt as to the interpretation of a pattern, contacting the clinician often results in a useful exchange whereby you learn that the patient has had chronic diarrhea and the clinician learns that the protein loss is severe enough to create a marked hypoalbuminemia. Such information is of further use in helping the clinician explain a corresponding lymphocytopenia, which may accompany protein loss in the gut [7].

Albumin is also often decreased, albeit to a lesser extent, in patients with acute inflammation and during chronic infections. By contrast, an elevated albumin indicates acute dehydration and is accompanied by an increase in the other serum proteins. Recently, we have seen several patients with normal or elevated albumin and decreased levels of the other serum proteins, which is a typical finding in patients who have been plasmapheresed for either therapy or donation and whose oncotic pressure has been stabilized by replacing their fluid with intravenous albumin.

ALPHA REGION

Alpha-1 Lipoprotein

Alpha-1 lipoprotein forms a very broad, usually rather faint band that extends through albumin into the alpha 1 zone (Figure 2-3). This band consists of high-density lipoproteins that may vary considerably in concentration in normal individuals as the result of diet as well as genetic differences (normal concentration, 250–390 mg/dl). Alpha-1 lipoproteins are absent in Tangier disease (inherited high-density lipoprotein deficiency) or may be decreased in a variety of conditions including chronic liver disease, renal disease, and with acute inflammation [9]. Elevated alpha-1 lipoprotein often reflects estrogen increase such as in pregnancy, with use of oral contraceptives, and in patients with cirrhosis [10].

Knowledge of this band is useful mainly for understanding its increase or decrease in a particular sample. Due to the variability of alpha-1 lipoproteins with normal samples and the diffuse nature of the band itself, the examination of this area alone is not particularly useful in diagnosis. Although it may be helpful when viewed with the entire pattern of the protein profile presented by HRE, one would not, for instance, refrain from interpreting a typical cirrhotic pattern as such merely because the alpha-1 lipoprotein was not elevated.

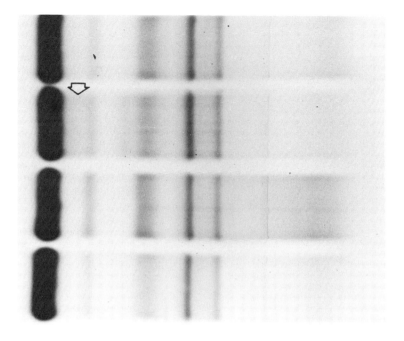

Figure 2-3. Alpha-1 lipoprotein is elevated in second sample from top. This produces a diffuse density (*arrow*) from albumin to the alpha-1 antitrypsin band.

Alpha-1 Antitrypsin

Alpha-1 antitrypsin is the major component of the discrete band in the alpha-1 region. Although it is represented by a relatively small band, in this text it is classified as a major protein band because of the clinical importance of associated abnormalities. The normal concentration of alpha-1 antitrypsin ranges from 100 to 400 mg/dl. Although its name implies that it functions to inhibit the activity of trypsin only, it interferes with the enzymatic activity of a variety of enzymes including trypsin, chymotrypsin, pancreatic elastase, skin collagenase, renin, urokinase, Hageman-factor cofactor, and leukocyte neutral proteases [11,12]. It is by far the most significant protease inhibitor in serum, accounting for more than 90% of the trypsin-inhibiting capacity of human serum [13].

Decreased Alpha-1 Antitrypsin

The most clinically significant finding on examining this band is decrease or absence, reflecting alpha-1 antitrypsin deficiency. The examiner must be extremely certain to inspect carefully the alpha-1 region of each electrophoretic strip for this possibility, as subtle decreases may be missed. The correlative use of densitometric scanning helps provide a double check, but may also provide a false sense of security. A borderline-normal densitometric scan (values in the low-but-normal range) does *not* rule out an alpha-1 antitrypsin deficiency. This may be due to a relatively large alpha-1 lipoprotein or may reflect the inherent inaccuracies of densitometric measurements of such small bands. The latter is reflected by our own studies showing a coefficient of variation of 10% for this region [14]. A low or decreased alpha-1 antitrypsin must be followed up by studies of the alpha-1 antitrypsin levels by quantitative or functional studies. When these are low, genetic studies should be done to provide prognostic information to the family [15,16]. Because of interference with quantification of alpha-1 antitrypsin levels by anticoagulants, serum should be used to measure the functional activity or the concentration by immune precipitation assays. However, either serum or plasma is suitable for phenotypic analysis by reference electrophoretic methods (starch block electrophoresis with immunofixation) [17].

Deficiency of alpha-1 antitrypsin is associated with severe lung and liver disease, presumably reflecting the unchecked endogenous activity of a variety of proteolytic enzymes that are continuously liberated by minor inflammatory events in these tissues. Early in life, affected individuals develop a form of cirrhosis characterized by large globules of amorphous periodic acid–Schiff-positive material that occur within the cytoplasm of hepatocytes in the periportal areas. These globules are distinguished from glycogen in that they are not digested by treatment with diastase. Immunohistochemical studies have shown this material to be an alpha-1 antitrypsin precursor that is not excreted [11,18,19] (Figure 2–4). In the lung, the relatively unchecked proteolytic activity due to the lack of alpha-1 antitrypsin results in early development of emphysema [20,21].

Alleles of Alpha-1 Antitrypsin

A complete discussion of the genetic polymorphism (involving about 30 possible alleles) of alpha-1 antitrypsin is beyond the scope of this volume, but some details are relevant to interpreting and understanding the HRE patterns that you will encounter in patients with alpha-1 antitrypsin deficiency. Expression of the two alleles of any individual is codominant, that is, each allele controls production of a specific alpha-1 antitrypsin molecule unaffected by the other allele. The alleles are referred to as Pi (standing for protease inhibitor) followed by a third letter characterizing the particular allele. A reasonable generalization is that the alpha-1 antitrypsin from alleles producing the lowest concentration has the slowest electrophoretic mobility.

The *most* common (hence, M) allele is PiM (Table 2–4), accounting for about 90% of most populations studied [22]. The most cathodal molecule, denoted by the letter Z, is associated with severe deficiency. About 3% of the United States population are phenotype PiMZ, which does not result in clinical deficiency (due to the PiM allele), while only 1 in 3630 is of the deficient PiZZ phenotype [11]. The second most common phenotype, referred to as S, electrophoretically migrates between M and Z. Individuals with PiSZ may also

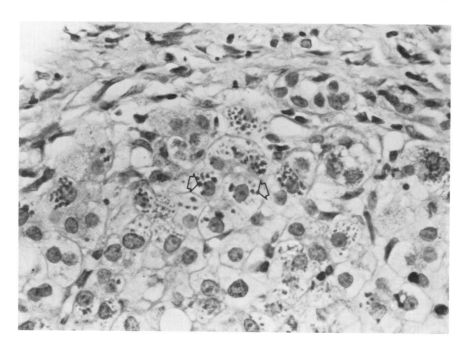

Figure 2-4. Liver from patient with alpha-1 antitrypsin deficiency (PiZZ) is depicted. The PAS, diastase stain, and digestion disclose the large granules (*arrows*), which are especially prominent in the periportal hepatocytes.

have clinically significant deficiency; this occurs in about 1 of 500 individuals in the United States [23].

In examining electrophoretic patterns, the most common genetic variant that the laboratorian will see is the PiMS banding (Figure 2-5). As with the PiMZ heterozygotes, these patients have no clinical disease, although there is obvious relevance for their progeny. The last allele likely to be detected by examination of HRE of serum is reflected by the protein product that migrates anodal to PiM and is termed PiF (fast). This genotype is not known to be associated with antitrypsin deficiency.

Table 2-4 Common Alpha-1

Phenotype	Antitrypsin Genotype	Phenotype Location	Normal Concentration (%)
PiM	MM	Mid-alpha-1	100
PiMS	MS	Mid- + slower alpha-1	80
PiS	SS	Slower alpha-1	60
PiMZ	MZ	Mid- + slowest alpha-1	60
PiZ	ZZ	Slowest alpha-1	15
PiF	FF	Anodal to M	—

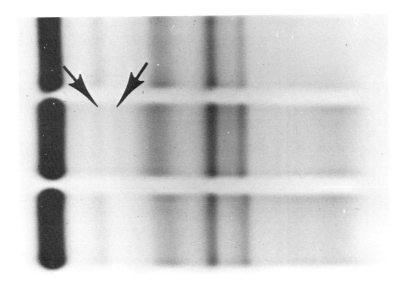

Figure 2-5. Middle serum is from patient with PiMS variant of alpha-1 antitrypsin. *Arrows* indicate the faintly staining bands. High-resolution electrophoresis (HRE) provides an excellent screening technique to pick up such abnormal patterns. Finding such a pattern should result in phenotypic analysis.

Most individuals who are heterozygous for deficiency phenotypes PiMZ, PiMS, and PiMF do not have an increased rate of chronic lung disease, although there has been some suggestion of an increased incidence of PiMZ among patients with lung disease [24]. Detailed studies of the variants that occur require more sophisticated methodologies than HRE [25], but HRE provides an excellent method to screen for the deficiency. When examining the HRE pattern one should be especially aware of samples with low and/or cathodally migrating alpha-1 bands (Figure 2-5). Again, clinical history (including age!) is important because premature infants, especially those with respiratory distress syndrome, often have decreased levels of alpha-1 antitrypsin that will recover with time. If the weak alpha-1 band is located in the slow alpha-1 region, you can suggest the possibility of PiZ, PiS, or PiSZ phenotypes, which has great clinical significance; large series have shown that the PiZ and PiSZ phenotypes may have hepatic dysfunction as early as the first 3 months of life [26].

Increased Alpha-1 Antitrypsin

Increased levels of alpha-1 antitrypsin occur in a variety of conditions and can be useful in pattern interpretations discussed later. Generally, it is increased as part of the acute phase response in patients with hyperestrogenemia due to pregnancy, oral contraceptives, or tumors, or with liver disease [27].

Note that the alpha-1 antitrypsin level will increase during an acute phase reaction even in patients with genetic deficiency of this protein. Therefore, in a patient suspected of having alpha-1 antitrypsin deficiency, normal levels of this protein do not in themselves rule out a deficiency. When we are quantifying alpha-1 antitrypsin in patients suspected of having a deficiency, we routinely quantify the C-reactive protein levels. When the C-reactive protein is elevated, a "normal" level of alpha-1 antitrypsin does not rule out the possibility of deficiency.

Alpha-1 Fetoprotein

Alpha-1 fetoprotein is present in neonatal serum in concentrations up to 40 mg/dl while normal adults have less than 1µg/dl [10]. Although this would never be seen on routine HRE, some patients with hepatocellular carcinoma have markedly elevated levels of this protein produced by the liver. In such cases an alpha-1 band may be detected [10].

Alpha-1 Acid Glycoprotein

Alpha-1 acid glycoprotein, also known as orosomucoid, is a minor band that occurs just anodal to alpha-1 antitrypsin. Although its serum concentration ranges from 50 to 150 mg/dl, it is usually not seen unless greatly elevated because its high sialic acid content interferes with binding of the Amido black or Coomassie blue used to stain the gels. The only signficant finding of this band relative to routine HRE interpretation is when it is increased to greater than 200 mg/dl; at this level, it may cause a blurring or a fuzzy appearance on the anodal side of alpha-1 antitrypsin [27]. Such an elevation is commonly seen with the acute phase reaction pattern and in uremic patients (this protein is normally lost through the glomerulus) [28,29]. Some clinicians believe that quantification of this protein is useful in detecting neonatal infections. Since the serum levels of orosomucoid are much lower at birth than in adults, levels of 60–80 mg/dl (normal adult) have been associated with neonatal sepsis [30,31]. These levels are too low, however, to be seen reliably by HRE and should be determined by immunochemical methods [32].

INTER-ALPHA-1, -ALPHA-2 REGION

A faint but distinct band or cluster of small bands is usually seen between the alpha-1 antitrypsin band and the densely staining alpha-2 region in normal samples (Figure 2–6). This is the sum of several components that occasionally may be seen as separate bands. Because the elevation, reduction, or slight alterations in the characteristics of these bands has little practical significance

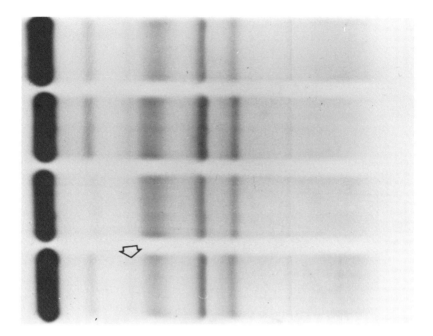

Figure 2-6. Small bands can often be seen in the inter-alpha-1, -alpha-2 region. They are particularly visible in top two and bottom samples (*arrow*).

for interpreting HRE patterns, we will only briefly review the responsible proteins.

Inter-Alpha-Trypsin Inhibitor

The most prominent of these proteins is inter-alpha-trypsin inhibitor, a 180,000-dalton protease inhibitor that represents 5% of the trypsin-inhibiting capability of normal serum. It is a precursor of a 30,000-dalton molecule that is an active protease inhibitor within the bronchial mucus and urine, sites where such inhibition may be critically important in preventing tissue damage [33].

Group-Specific Component

Group-specific component (Gc) is another protein responsible for this faint region in normal individuals. Gc is the protein product of a polymorphic gene that has proven useful in paternity testing because of the different patterns seen by isoelectric focusing [34,35]. In some systems this migrates more cathodally, nearer to the transferrin band. Gc proteins are known to serve as carrier protein for vitamin D^3 metabolites and recently has been found to bind to the monomeric globular form of actin [36] and to cell-membrane-associated immunoglobulins [37]. The association with actin is seen clinically in pregnancy; when quantities of actin are released from trophoblast cells, the Gc protein has been shown to serve as a scavenger to bind this released actin [38]. However, as with other proteins in this category, accurate measurement requires means other than HRE.

Pregnancy Zone Protein

Another protein present in this region is the pregnancy zone protein, also known as pregnancy-associated alpha-2 glycoprotein. During pregnancy, this large glycoprotein (430,000 daltons) increases from less than 0.5 to 2 mg/dl [39]. The faint band(s) in this region also increase during acute inflammation [40–42]. As with most minor bands, current HRE techniques are not useful to demonstrate a reduction in the specific components.

Haptoglobin

Haptoglobin is an alpha-migrating protein that binds free hemoglobin liberated during intravascular hemolysis. During this process, the haptoglobin attaches to the globin portion of the hemoglobin molecule. The resulting haptoglobin–hemoglobin complex is rapidly taken up by the reticuloendothelial system, where the iron is liberated for reuse. This haptoglobin–hemoglobin complex is removed at the rate of 15 mg/100 ml/hour. Therefore, intravascular hemolysis usually is associated with decreased haptoglobin rather than free hemoglobin, unless there has been recent massive hemolysis [40].

On HRE, haptoglobin has a relatively complex pattern that often causes confusion about what is happening in the alpha-2 region. This complexity results from genetic polymorphism and the alteration of electrophoretic mobility by the haptoglobin-hemoglobin complex; the latter most commonly due to improper handling of blood specimens, but may be seen with recent massive hemolysis.

Three major phenotypes of haptoglobin can be discerned by the HRE pattern (Table 2–5). Haptoglobin type 1-1 is found in individuals who are homozygous for the Hp1 allele [41]. Its name reflects the fact that it has the

Table 2–5   Characteristics of the Major Haptoglobulin Phenotypes[a]

Haptoglobin Phenotype	Molecular Weight	HRE Migration
Hp type 1–1	80,000	Mid-alpha 1 to alpha 2
Hp type 2–1	120,000	Mid-alpha 2
Hp type 2–2	160,000	Slow alpha 2

Source: Data from Janik [10].

fastest electrophoretic mobility, migrating anodal to alpha-2 macroglobulin and obscuring the minor inter-alpha-trypsin inhibitor region bands. The cathodal end of this haptoglobin type merges with alpha-2 macroglobulin, preventing complete separation of these two proteins by HRE. About 10–15% of the population have this phenotype. Haptoglobin type 1-2 is slower than type 1-1, is heavier, and is usually present in a greater concentration in the serum (Table 2–5). It migrates directly over alpha-2 macroglobulin with its anodal end often meeting the small inter-alpha-trypsin inhibitor region. The third major phenotype of haptoglobin is slow-migrating type 2-2, a molecule twice the size of type 1-1 (Table 2–5) that is cathodal to alpha-2 macroglobulin. Unfortunately, although these three types represent the major types of haptoglobin, many variants exist that shift the migration slightly and cause unpredictable migration patterns that can be frustrating when trying to interpret the alpha-2 region [43,44].

Decreased Haptoglobin

Several important causes of decreased haptoglobin levels can be suggested by the HRE pattern (Table 2–6); the most clinically significant causes relate to hemolysis. For the clinician studying a patient with a hemolytic process, the laboratory interpretation of "marked decrease in haptoglobin consistent with intravascular hemolysis" is useful both in defining the process (extravascular for the individual sample) and in following the response of the patient to therapy. As usual, there are some caveats. An uncommon phenotypic variant of

---

Table 2-6   Decreased Haptoglobin

Hemolysis

In vivo:

Intravascular hemolysis
Extravascular hemolysis

In vitro:

Poor blood sampling technique;
  (hemoglobin–haptoglobin migrates
  cathodally near transferrin)

Ineffective erythropoiesis

Vitamin B_{12} deficiency
Folate deficiency

Congenital

HpO phenotype

Neonates

Normally have low haptoglobin

---

haptoglobin, referred to as type 0-0, produces no or very low levels of haptoglobin. Further, infants have little haptoglobin; the concentration goes from virtually zero in the cord blood to adult levels by around 4 months of age [40]. Ineffective erythropoiesis such as occurs during folate and B_{12} deficiency also gives rise to a noticeable decrease in the haptoglobin region of the HRE.

As with many conditions, the laboratorian must be given pertinent clinical information to be of optimal assistance in correct interpretation of the HRE patterns. When we find a markedly decreased haptoglobin and no clinical information is provided, we should share this information with the clinician and request pertinent information such as: "Is the patient an infant? Does the patient have an autoimmune disorder or symptoms suggesting this (many are associated with intravascular hemolysis)? Has the patient had a recent blood transfusion? Is there a known hereditary anemia (sickle cell or thalassemia) in this patient's family? Is the patient taking any drugs that may be associated with increased intravascular hemolysis? Has the patient had cardiac surgery? Does the patient have symptoms consistent with malaria or other infections associated with intravascular hemolysis? Do the red blood cell indices suggest a megaloblastic anemia?"

Perhaps my list is too long (or too short), but it may serve to emphasize the key role that the laboratorian can play in shortening a patient's hospital stay and in streamlining the diagnostic process by guiding clinicians when significant HRE data is related to pertinent clinical information. Although HRE does not give sufficient resolution to distinguish between type 1-2 and type 2-2 haptoglobin variants (isoelectric focusing or starch gel electrophoresis is needed for such phenotypic analysis), it does allow one to recognize elevations or reductions that provide clinically useful information.

A decrease in haptoglobin may reflect intravascular hemolysis, ineffective erythropoiesis, or the uncommon congential hypohaptoglobinemia seen most frequently in Blacks [45]. When hemoglobin binds to haptoglobin, the complex has a much slower migration than that of haptoglobin alone (Figure 2–7). The pattern shown in Figure 2–7 usually indicates that the sample has been handled poorly with *in vitro* hemolysis producing the haptoglobin-hemoglobin band indicated. However, in cases of recent incompatible blood transfusion or recent massive hemolysis, as in malaria or clostridial infections, this may reflect an urgent clinical situation. Once again, clinical information is the critical ingredient for correct interpretation.

Increased Haptoglobin

An increased synthesis of haptoglobin occurs in patients with an acute inflammatory response and in patients with increased estrogen stimulation (pregnancy, contraceptive drugs, estrogen-secreting neoplasms, and cirrhosis). A given patient may have simultaneous processes that result in a normal haptoglobin HRE pattern when an elevation or decrease may have been predicted by the available clinical information. For instance, if a patient has an autoim-

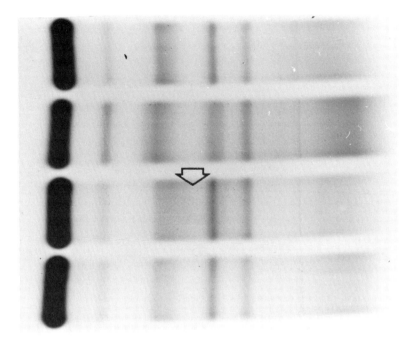

Figure 2-7. Top sample is from patient with the most common type 1-2 haptoglobin. The second sample has more anodal migration seen in the alpha-2 region because it is from a patient with type 1-1 haptoglobin. The third sample was hemolyzed and shows the cathodal slurring that results from the hemoglobin–haptoglobin complex (*arrow*).

mune disease with intravascular hemolysis, the haptoglobin should be decreased. However, if the autoimmune disease is clinically active with acute inflammation, there will be a stimulation of haptoglobin production by the liver. In this case, the haptoglobin shown by HRE will depend on which process predominated at the time the sample was taken [46].

Alpha-2 Macroglobulin

Alpha-2 macroglobulin is the other major protein migrating in the alpha-2 region. With a concentration of 175–400 mg/dl, it accounts for about 3% of the total proteins in serum [47]. Due to the variable migration of the haptoglobin types, alpha-2 macroglobulin is not often seen as a discrete band. An important exception is the neonate, in whom little haptoglobin is present and alpha-2 macroglobulin levels are much higher than in adults (Figure 2-8). Alpha-2 macroglobulin is an enormous molecule with a molecular weight of 800,000 and a sedimentation coefficient of 19 S that functions primarily as a

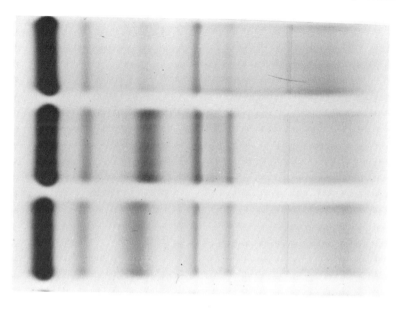

Figure 2-8. Top serum is from patient with hemolytic anemia and an extremely low haptoglobin. The alpha-2 region protein seen is alpha-2 macroglobulin. Middle sample is from a pregnant woman with an increase in alpha-1, alpha-2, and transferrin (the beta-1 band).

protease inhibitor. While it is particularly effective at inhibiting plasmin activity [48], alpha-2 macroglobulin is also able to inhibit the enzymes trypsin, chymotrypsin, thrombin, and elastase. It is also the major serum collagenase inhibitor, which may be important in preventing lung damage during pneumonitis when there is considerable local collagenase activity [49,50].

Alpha-2 macroglobulin is elevated in neonates, the elderly, patients with elevated estrogen levels, and especially as part of the nephrotic pattern (see following section) in patients with selective glomerular leakage. In several forms of alpha-1 antitrypsin deficiency (PiZ, PiMZ, and other rare variants), most patients who have emphysema have an increased concentration of alpha-2 macroglobulin. As such it may reflect a protective response to the increased inflammatory injury occurring in these patients [51]. An elevated alpha-2 macroglobulin can usually be seen as a sharp increase in the anodal end of the alpha-2 globulin region (Figure 2-8), but may be masked by an elevated or even a high-normal level of haptoglobin.

A decrease in alpha-2 macroglobulin is extremely difficult to detect by using HRE. Haptoglobin will almost always hinder such an interpretation. Therefore, although a decreased alpha-2 macroglobulin is associated with a variety of clinical conditions such as hyaline membrane disease, rheumatoid arthritis, disseminated intravascular coagulation, multiple myeloma, and peptic ulcer disease, you will not be able to detect this on HRE gels.

Ceruloplasmin

Ceruloplasmin is an important copper-binding transport protein that may increase during an acute phase reaction. However, its low concentration in normal serum precludes its detection on the routine serum protein electrophoresis. Even during the acute phase response it is difficult to see because of the increase in the other alpha-2 globulins. It is known to be elevated in the acute phase response, in steroid therapy, and in cases of biliary tract obstruction.

The most significant feature of ceruloplasmin is its marked decrease in patients with Wilson's disease. The lack of this transport protein is thought to play the major role in hepatolenticular degeneration. However, HRE will not aid in the detection of a decreased ceruloplasmin; specific assays must be performed.

Prebeta Lipoprotein

HRE is not used to screen for lipid abnormalities; however, some patients will have unusual patterns due to hyperlipidemia. In the prebeta area, a broad elevation like that seen with hemolysis also occurs in patients with elevated prebeta lipoprotein (Figure 2-9). Therefore, when we see an elevation in this area, we look for hemolyzed serum. If it is not, we suggest lipoprotein electrophoresis.

Alpha-1 Antichymotrypsin

Alpha-1 antichymotrypsin is another protein found in the alpha-1–alpha-2 interregion. It is about one-tenth as prominent as the alpha-1 antitrypsin band with a serum concentration of 30–60 mg/dl and a molecular weight of 69,000, and has only weak protease inhibitor function. Although its name implies a role in chymotrypsin inhibition, it probably provides less significant inhibition than does alpha-1 antitrypsin [39]. In serum, its concentration increases rapidly after acute injury, especially in thermal injury, perhaps acting to inhibit some of the enzymes liberated during this process [40]. By HRE, one only sees a variable, deeper staining in the alpha-1–alpha-2 interregion. Obviously, a decreased alpha-1 antichymotrypsin concentration would not be detectable by the HRE techniques described here.

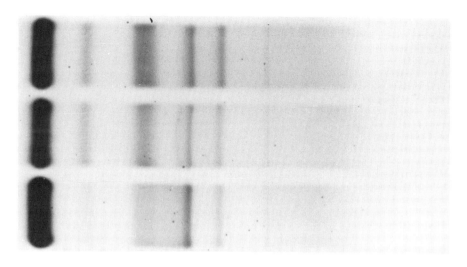

Figure 2-9. Bottom sample is from patient with marked elevation in prebeta lipo-protein. The strip looks like the hemolyzed serum pattern. When such a pattern is seen, the serum should be examined for the differential.

Cold-Insoluble Globulin

Cold-insoluble globulin (fibronectin) is a faint band regularly seen between the alpha-2 and beta-1 regions. It is a large, 350,000-dalton protein that derived its original name from the observation that it precipitates in the cold and in heparin. The band becomes more prominent during pregnancy or with cholestasis when the protein increases beyond its usual serum range of 15–30 mg/dl [10]. Recent studies have demonstrated that fibronectin acts in the wound healing process by mediating the adherence of fibroblasts and monocytes at sites of tissue damage [41]. During the first 48 hours of the acute inflammatory response, fibronectin is rapidly deposited in the damaged tissue. Simultaneously, its concentration in the serum decreases [41].

BETA REGION

Transferrin

Transferrin is the next major band at the beginning of the beta region. It is a useful landmark in patients who have complicated alpha-2 regions because of genetic variants or hemolysis. Transferrin has a molecular weight of 80,000 and functions to transport nonheme free iron from the gastrointestinal tract to the bone marrow. Each transferrin molecule can bind two molecules of free iron, but normally only about one-third of the transferrin molecules are saturated with iron. The total iron binding capacity of serum is a reflection of the amount of transferrin present; its normal concentration is 200–400 mg/dl. In patients with iron-deficiency anemia, the levels of transferrin are considerably increased. Determination of the transferrin levels is useful in distinguishing between iron-deficiency anemia (inadequate intake or chronic hemorrhage with loss of iron stores) from iron-refractory anemias. In iron deficiency, the concentration of serum transferrin goes up, but as less iron is available for transport, the saturation of the transferrin falls, often to less than 15% as compared to a normal of 33%. Transferrin levels are also increased in patients with hyperestrogen secretion.

As it is synthesized in the liver, transferrin usually appears at a decreased level in chronic liver disease. During acute inflammation the synthesis of transferrin is largely shut down, resulting in a faint beta-1 band (Chapter 3). Transferrin is also decreased during renal disease and thermal injuries due to loss through the glomeruli and damaged skin, respectively [45].

HRE is useful in distinguishing relatively common genetic variants of transferrin (Figure 2–10). Both electrophoretically slow and fast variants of transferrin have been identified. Homozygotes are rarely seen, perhaps because they would be difficult to recognize by HRE techniques; however, heterozygotes are easily seen as two equal staining bands in the beta-1 region.

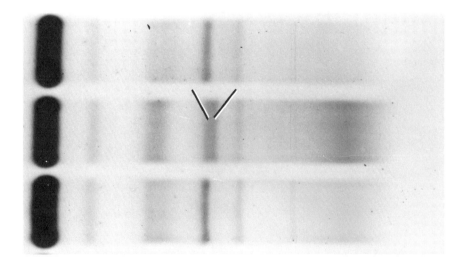

Figure 2–10. Middle serum is from patient with genetic variant of transferrin. There are two discrete bands (*indicated*) of equivalent intensity. It is important to know of this variant to avoid mistaking it for complement activation or a monoclonal protein migrating in the beta-1 region.

These represent the codominant expression of two alleles, one normal and one variant [2]. These variants have no known functional effect on patients. It is important to understand how the genetic variants look, however, as other clinically signficant lines can appear in this area and must be distinguished from the transferrin variants.

Beta-Migrating Monoclonal Gammopathies and Complement Activation Products

The major proteins that need to be distinguished from the double transferrin line are beta-migrating monoclonal gammopathies and complement activation products. It is often erroneously believed that immunoglobulin molecules only migrate in the gamma region. Although IgG is predominantly in the gamma region, IgM tends to stay around the origin and IgA is *mainly* a beta-migrating molecule. Further, the uncommon IgD and the more common light chain monoclonals (Bence Jones protein) will frequently occur in the beta or even in the alpha globulin regions. Therefore, a distortion of the beta-1 transferrin area must be inspected carefully. Monoclonal proteins of the IgA type will be denser and more diffuse than the equal transferrin lines seen in the heterozygous variants (Figure 2–11). Again, this is a situation in which some clinical history will help guide interpretation. If the patient has any symptoms compatible with a monoclonal gammopathy, quantification of the serum immunoglobulins will determine its presence. An IgA monoclonal band large enough

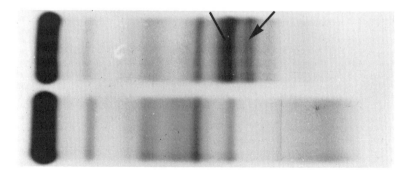

Figure 2–11. Top sample is typical of IgA monoclonal protein. Note extra, dense-staining beta-region band (*indicated*), which may be mistaken for a transferrin variant. When identification is uncertain, IgA quantification will reveal an elevated IgA. The extra, faintly staining band just anodal to the origin (*arrow*) represents the polymeric form of this same monoclonal protein. Its migration could cause confusion with fibrinogen in an incompletely clotted sample.

to be seen in the beta region would give a significant elevation of IgA by quantification. Also, if Bence Jones protein is suspected, immunoanalysis of the urine would be useful.

The other major protein band of clinical significance that is often confused with the transferrin variant is the C3c split product of complement. This may be an *in vitro* activation from poor specimen handling or may reflect *in vivo* activation caused by autoimmune disease or ongoing inflammation. This activation can be identified by immunofixation performed on the serum specimen. A discussion with the clinician and analysis of a fresh specimen will help distinguish a reflection of real disease from a laboratory handling problem.

Beta Lipoprotein

Beta lipoprotein (low-density lipoprotein) is an unusual molecule in two respects: its position varies considerably depending on its concentration, and it has an irregular anodal front (Figure 2-12). The molecular weight is an enormous 2,400,000, and its concentration spans the wide gap between 200 and 700 mg/dl. Beta lipoprotein serves to transport lipids, cholesterol, and hormones. Because the migration of beta lipoprotein decreases with increasing concentration, it may be found anodal to the transferrin band or cathodal to the C3 band. This self-slowing process with an irregular anodal front also occurs with IgM and IgA monoclonal gammopathies. It is related to the tendency of these molecules to aggregate when present in high concentration. At the anodal edge, the movement is faster and the concentration of the molecules is lower than at the center of the band where aggregation tends to occur. The aggregation of these large molecules interferes with the electrical field and endosmotic flow (see Chapter 1) in the immediate vicinity of the band. The partial interruption of the regular electrical field and endosmotic flow results in an irregular band or small parallel bands (striae) with a crescentic shape, the middle lagging toward the cathode [47]. Such irregularity is especially pronounced in gels that have narrower pores with a greater molecular sieve capability (Figure 2-12). While such gels often give excellent resolution of gamma globulins, the beta lipoprotein band can obscure the other important beta proteins. Elevated levels of beta lipoprotein are seen in conditions with increased cholesterol such as the nephrotic syndrome and Type II hypercholesterolemia.

C3

After transferrin, C3, the third component of complement, is the next major protein band (Figure 2-13) and the only component of complement that can be readily recognized by HRE. It is a large molecule (180,000 daltons) that is normally present in serum at a concentration of 55–180 mg/dl. This band's density and position can vary depending on genetic differences, active inflam-

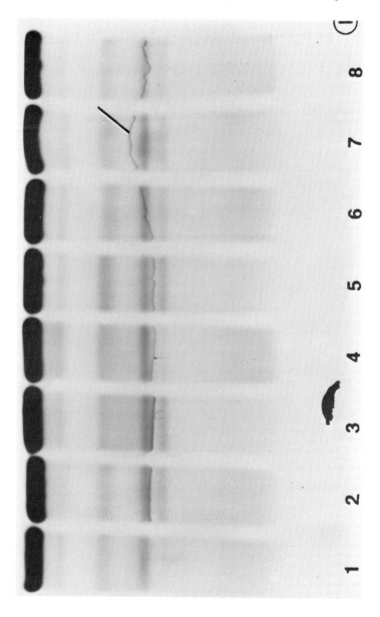

Figure 2–12.   The irregular beta-lipoprotein bands (*indicated* for second sample from top) are especially obvious on this gel.

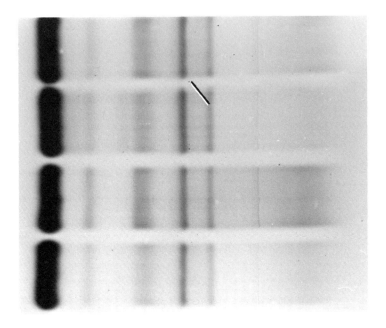

Figure 2-13. The C3 band (indicated in second sample from top) is the next major band following transferrin in most HRE gels.

matory disease, or poor specimen processing. A detailed discussion of complement activation is beyond the scope of this volume, and excellent reviews are available [52]. However, it is worth giving the reader a few basic details that have relevance for understanding changes seen in the major protein band on HRE.

Classic Pathway of Complement Activation

Complement is a complex series of serum proteins that may be activated by the interactions of antibody with antigen or by a variety of other stimuli (Table 2-7). C3 may be decreased when either the classical or alternative pathway is activated. In the classical pathway (Table 2-8), C1q must attach to one of the activating factors listed in Table 2-7. Then, in the presence of calcium, C1q forms a stable molecular complex with C1r and C1s. During this process, C1r is activated to a proteolytic form that cleaves C1s to $\overline{C1s}$ (a pivotal esterase in the complement activation sequence). During small inflammatory responses, this C1 esterase will be inactivated by C1 esterase inhibitor. Deficiency of the C1 esterase inhibitor can result in an overwhelming complement activation following a relatively trivial inciting inflammation. Patients with deficiency of C1 esterase inhibitor develop bouts of angioedema locally at the

Table 2–7   Factors That Activate Complement

Classical Pathway	Alternative Pathway
Immune complexes	Aggregated immunoglobulin
Staphylococcal protein A-1gG	Complex polysaccharides:
Polyanions:	Bacterial dextrans
DNA	Inulin
Dextran sulfate	Erythrocyte stroma
Some RNA viruses	Cobra venom factor
C-Reactive protein	Nephritic factor

Table 2–8   Sequence of Complement Activation in the Classical Pathway

Activator	Factor(s)	Activated Product	Circulating Split Products
1. Classical pathway activator (CPA)	C1q		
2. C1q–CPA	C1r, C1s (with Ca^{++})	C1qrs	
3. C1$\overline{qrs}$[a]–CPA	C4	C4b	C4a
4. C4b–C1$\overline{qrs}$–CPA	C2	C2a	
5. C2a C4b[b]	C3	C3b	C3a
6. C3b,C2a,C46	C5	C5b	C5a
7. C5b	C6,C7,C8,C9	Lysis	

[a]The bar over components indicates that they are in an activated state that functions as a proteolytic enzyme for the next component in the system.
[b]Only one of the many C2a,C4b (C3 convertase) complexes created by Activator #4 is shown.

site of the complement activation. When such activity involves the oropharynx, the process can be fatal.

When $\overline{\text{C1s}}$ is not inactivated, it cleaves C4 into C4b (195,000 daltons), which attaches to the initiating complex, and a smaller 10,000-dalton C4a fragment that may attach to nearby mast cells. Next, C2 is cleaved by the same $\overline{\text{C1s}}$ into a small C2b and a larger (80,000) C2a fragment. The latter fragment attaches to C4b, giving the C3 convertase complex C2a,C4b. Multiple C3 convertase complexes can be created by one C1qrs complex. This is a major amplification step in the complement activation process.

C3 convertase cleaves native C3 into the small, active molecule C3a and a larger C3b fragment (Figure 2–14). C3a is a particularly active 9,000-dalton polypeptide. It can induce vasodilatation and increase vascular permeability with resulting edema. The presence of C3b on the initiating complex has func-

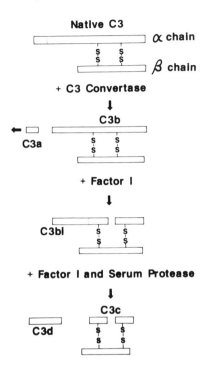

Figure 2-14.   Schematic representation of C3 activation.

tional significance. Most phagocytic cells have receptors for C3b on their surfaces, and, therefore, the C3b on the surface of the initiating complex will be more readily attached to neutrophils, monocytes, and eosinophils.

Together, C3b,C2a,C4b constitutes C5 convertase, which is the active complex that begins the terminal phase of complement activation by cleaving C5 into C5a and C5b. Once again, the smaller C5a polypeptide has important biologic activities. In addition to causing vasodilatation and increased vascular permeability as C3a, C5a is chemotactic for neutrophils and monocytes and can attach to mast cells. Together, C3a and C5a are referred to as *anaphylatoxins*.

After C5b attaches to the membrane of the cell at or near the initiating complex, it provides the site where C6, C7, C8, and C9 attach. The C5-9 complex creates a disturbance in the structural integrity of the membrane by forming a pore or channel with resultant lysis.

Alternative Pathway of Complement Activation

The alternative pathway of complement activation can be triggered by a variety of substances in the absence of a specific antibody–antigen interaction

(Table 2–7). The key to the system is an alternative method to form C5 convertase, which will trigger the remainder of the complement components. This pathway depends on the continuous reaction of C3 with properdin Factor B in the presence of Mg^{++} with formation of C3,B complex (Table 2–9). The latter is rapidly cleaved by Factor D to form C3,Bb. Because C3,Bb is only weakly proteolytic for C3, small amounts of C3b and C3a are generated. When no appropriate activating surface is present (Table 2–7), Factor H quickly binds to C3b, preventing its association with Factor B. Also, Factor I together with Factor H can inactivate C3b. When an activating surface such as bacterial polysaccharides is present, C3b can react with Factor B to yield C3b,B. Once again, the B portion of the complex is cleaved by Factor D resulting in the formation of C3b,Bb. As a negative feedback to prevent overactivation by trivial insults, Factor H promotes dissociation of the complex.

When sufficient C3b,Bb is produced to overcome the suppressive effects of Factors H and I, the C3b,Bb complex is stabilized by reacting with properdin forming C3b,Bb,P. The latter is a C5 convertase, which begins the terminal activation of the complement components.

During inactivation of C3b, Factor I first cleaves the alpha chain into the inactive C3bi (Figure 2–14). Next, in a kinetically slower reaction, Factor I cleaves the terminal end of the alpha chain, resulting in the formation of a small C3d fragment (30,000) and a larger C3c fragment (160,000) that is often seen in HRE of poorly processed blood samples or aged specimens. In the latter reaction, Factor I collaborates with serum proteases. C3c is readily seen in HRE patterns, usually with a decreased or absent C3 band (Figure 2–15). Usually, the presence of the C3c band indicates that the specimen has been processed poorly, stored at room temperature, lyophilized (most lyophilized commericial standard serum preparations will show this C3c band), or stored for several days at 4°C (Figure 2–16). Due to the short biologic half-life of

Table 2–9 Sequence of Complement Activation in the Alternative Pathway

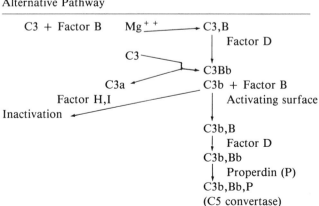

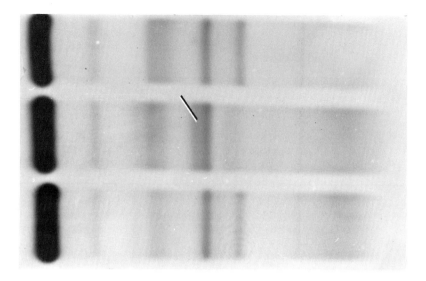

Figure 2–15. C3 activation is seen in middle sample. A C3c band is now present (indicated), while the C3 band is slurred toward the anode.

C3c, it is unlikely that the C3c seen by HRE relates to active inflammation *in vivo*.

C4

In some patients with an acute inflammatory reaction, C4 may be seen just anodal to C3. The normal serum concentration of C4 is 15–50 mg/dl. Knowing the position of this band is relevant primarily to the possibility of a beta-migrating monoclonal protein. If the serum IgA level is in the normal range and the patient has an obvious acute phase pattern (Chapter 3), quantification of serum C4 will quickly explain the nature of the band.

Fibrinogen

Although fibrinogen is not present in properly processed normal serum, a small fibrinogen band is often seen in serum protein electrophoresis due to insufficient clotting or failure to remove the serum from the clot with the release of fibrinogen breakdown products (Figure 2–17). Fibrinogen may also be seen in the "serum" of patients on heparin therapy. It is strongly recommended that plasma not be used for HRE study as the fibrinogen band obscures an important part of the beta-gamma area. Since the single most important find-

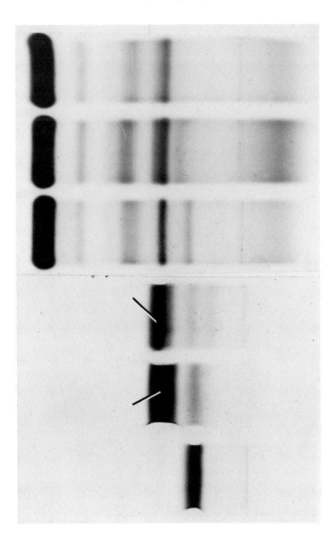

Figure 2-16. Top three samples show a lyophilized control specimen, serum from a patient with systemic lupus erythematosus (SLE) with activation of complement, and a serum with normal C3. The three samples are repeated in an immunofixation study in which C3 and C3 products are precipitated by a specific antiserum to C3. Note the major product seen in both lyophilized serum and that from patient with SLE has anodal migration (*indicated*). These bands stain considerably denser than native serum because the immunoglobulin reagent enhances sensitivity by its contribution to the protein staining.

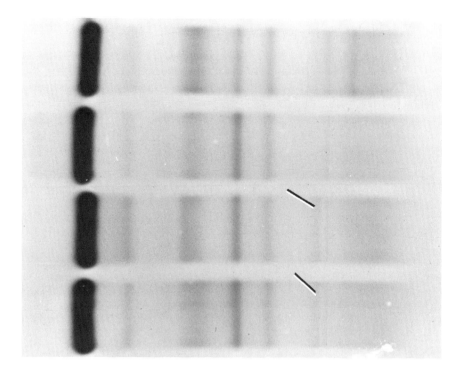

Figure 2-17.   A faintly staining fibrinogen band just anodal to the origin is best seen in the bottom two samples (*indicated*), although it is also present in the top sample. This is usually due to incomplete clotting of a specimen. One might mistake this for a monoclonal band. Typically, however, most of the samples from a day's run will have this artifact. When only a single specimen shows this band, we repeat the sample after complete clotting to insure that a monoclonal band is not present.

ing that can be made by HRE study of a sample is the presence of a monoclonal gammopathy, the presence of fibrinogen in a sample is deleterious to that determination.

GAMMA REGION

C-Reactive Protein

C-Reactive protein is a 135,000-dalton nonimmunoglobulin protein that migrates in the gamma region. C-Reactive protein derives its name from the fact that it reacts with the capsular polysaccharide of *Streptococcus pneumoniae* [53]. Recently, it has been found to be one of the most reliable, objective measures of the acute inflammatory response [54]. As with most of the bands discussed above, its exact position will vary somewhat depending on the particular electrophoretic system being used. Although its normal concentration of <2 mg/dl is far too low to be noticed, it may increase considerably during acute inflammatory responses to levels greater than 100 mg/dl. In the latter, it creates a distinctive midgamma band that looks exactly like a small monoclonal protein (Figure 2–18). Since the elevation of C-reactive protein occurs during an acute inflammatory response, the presence of the typical acute phase pattern (Chapter 3) should alert the reader to include C-reactive protein in the differential. Quantification of C-reactive protein level or immunofixation for C-reactive protein (Chapter 4) is required to achieve correct identification of the restricted area.

Immunoglobulins

The gamma region consists almost entirely of immunoglobulin molecules. Because of the relatively slow migration of most of these molecules, the term "gamma globulin" was at one time synonymous with immunoglobulin. It is now clear that antibody molecules migrate anywhere from the alpha region

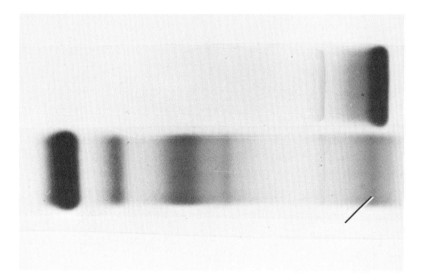

Figure 2–18. The C-reactive protein was markedly elevated and resulted in a subtle but discrete band (*indicated*) in the midgamma region. To demonstrate the true nature of this band, antiserum specific for C-reactive protein was used in the immunofixation shown immediately above the sample. Note that this serum is from a patient with an acute phase reaction and shows increased alpha-1, alpha-2, and decreased transferrin. The C3 band is missing because sample had been stored for several days before immunofixation for this demonstration.

through the slow gamma area. The orginal term *gamma globulin* referred to the fact that most of the serum antibodies are of the IgG class, which primarily migrates in a gamma location.

To understand the unusually broad electrophoretic migration of this important group of molecules, it is worth reviewing briefly the structure of immunoglobulin. (More detailed reviews of structure can be found elsewhere [55].) The basic monomeric unit of an immunoglobulin molecule consists of two identical heavy polypeptide chains and two identical light polypeptide chains (Figure 2–19). One reason for the vast heterogeneity of pI among immunoglobulins is that there are five different major classes of immunoglobulin heavy chains and two different classes of immunoglobulin light chains; each has different electrophoretic mobilities. Additionally, there are millions of possible antigen-combining sites in the Fab region, creating an enormous diversity of charge.

The characteristics of the heavy chain bands are listed in Table 2–10. Immunoglobulin molecules are named for their heavy chain class, which is of major importance in the biologic capabilities of the molecule (Table 2–10). The five major classes of immunoglobulins are IgG, IgA, IgM, IgD, and IgE. Any heavy chain may be combined with either of the two light chain types, kappa or lambda. The normal kappa/lambda ratio is 2:1.

During early studies of the basic molecular structure of immunoglobulins, it was found that the enzyme papain would cleave the molecule into two major fragments. One fragment was called Fc (the fragment that crystallized), while the other fragment was called Fab (the fragment with antigen-binding activity) (Figure 2–19). Fc was found to be the C-terminal half of the two heavy chains, and Fab contains an intact light chain and the N-terminal half of one heavy chain. Further investigation into amino acid sequences of the immunoglobulins took advantage of the fact that myeloma proteins provide extremely large amounts of a single, specific immunoglobulin molecule. These studies disclosed that the C-terminal half of all kappa light chains is remarkably homogeneous (constant region) while the N-terminal half varies considerably from one kappa light chain protein to another (variable region).

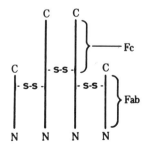

Figure 2–19. Schematic representation of the immunoglobulin molecule.

Table 2-10 Characteristics of Human Immunoglobulins

Characteristics	IgG	IgA	IgM	IgD	IgE
Concentration[a]	600–1600	25–390	20–390	—	—
Molecular weight	160,000	160,000–350,000	200,000–900,000	170,000	190,000
Complement activation	+	±	+ +	0	0
Opsonization	+	0	0	0	0
Secretory	0	+	+	0	0
Cross placenta	+	0	0	0	0
Binds mast cell	0	0	0	0	+
Membrane Ig	±	±	+	+	—

[a]Concentration in mg/dl.

Similarly, the N-terminal fourth of a gamma heavy chain (variable region) varies in amino acid composition from one myeloma protein to another, while the C-terminal three-fourths (constant region) are almost identical. Obviously, there is a relationship between the variable heavy and light chain region and the specific antigen-binding function of the N terminus of the molecule.

There is occasional confusion about nomenclature of immunoglobulins. *Isotype* refers to the heavy chain class; therefore, there are five major isotypes—IgG, IgA, IgM, IgD, and IgE. The term *idiotype* refers to the specific antigenic makeup of the variable portion of the Fab region; this is unique to an antibody molecule of a certain specificity. I like to oversimplify and think of the "idiotype" as referring to the specific binding site of the antibody molecule. *Allotype* refers to certain genetic alleles that may occur within the population such as Gm1 or Gm2.

The Fc portion of the immunoglobulin molecule determines the biologic capabilities of the antibody. For instance, IgG1, IgG3, and IgG4 have Fc regions that are capable of activating complement via the classical pathway following an antibody–antigen interaction. IgA and IgG2 are relatively ineffective at complement activation due to the structure of their Fc regions. The biologic activities of antibodies listed in Table 2–10 depend almost entirely on the Fc region.

IgG

IgG, the major immunoglobulin occupying the gamma region, is responsible for this diffuse, light-staining region in normal individuals. In adults, IgG occurs in a concentration of 600–1600 mg/dl, whereas in children the concentration is variable. Neonates will have almost normal adult levels, as this molecule is transported across the placenta via specific Fc receptors on the placenta. However, the newborn child does not synthesize IgG in adult quantities for several months. The maternal IgG that crossed the placenta is gradually catabolized so that at about six months a nadir is reached where extremely low levels of IgG are present in the serum. One of the main reasons that children with congenital immunodeficiencies are asymptomatic until after six months of age is the protection afforded them by their maternal IgG.

Many abnormalities of IgG occur. Elevations with infections, autoimmune diseases, liver disease, and myeloma are commonly seen. Peculiar patterns such as those due to immune complexes or oligoclonal patterns are found in the gamma region. Decrease in IgG demonstrated by finding faint staining of the gamma region is a highly significant pattern that must be pursued clinically. These pattern diagnoses are discussed in detail in Chapter 3.

IgM

IgM usually occurs as a pentamer in the serum. As such, it has a molecular weight of about 1,000,000, and the normal concentration is 20–390 mg/dl. It is the most effective of all isotypes in activating complement. Whereas IgG may require 100 or more molecules in an antibody-antigen complex to effectively activate complement, a single IgM molecule will suffice for complete activation through the terminal lytic sequence on a cell surface. This property probably relates not only to the amino acid makeup of the Fc portion, but also to the physical proximity of the five Fc groups of the pentamar. IgM is such a bulky molecule that it does not stray too far from the origin of HRE. Depending on the character of the support medium for the particular HRE system (see Chapter 1), it may migrate slightly cathodally or slightly anodally. By HRE, IgM is not normally visible other than as a faint haze around the origin. Marked elevations, which may occur with infections or malignancy, are reviewed further in Chapter 3.

IgA

IgA, the other major isotype of immunoglobulin in the serum, occurs mainly as a 7 S monomer that weighs 160,000 daltons and has a concentration of 25–390 mg/dl. IgA is thought to function mainly along mucosal surfaces where it is the most prominent immunoglobulin isotype [56]. Along the mucosa of the gastrointestinal tract, respiratory tract, or mammary or other glands, IgA is secreted from the plasma cells as a dimer attached by a small 12,000-polypeptide called a joining chain. It then migrates toward the surface epithelium (Figure 2–20) where it combines with a 60,000-dalton glycoprotein called secretory component, which is made by the surface epithelium. This is secreted into the mucosal lumen where it probably functions to prevent pathogenic microorganisms and their toxic products from entering and attaching to the surface epithelium. IgA is a poor activator of complement and does not opsonize for phagocytosis. Its role in the serum is unclear, although some recent studies suggest it may be able to collaborate with killer cells in cytotoxic reactions.

Isolated IgA deficiency is the most common of all immunodeficiencies, occurring in 1 of 700 individuals. Although there is usually a compensatory increase of IgM along the mucosal surfaces, these patients have a significantly increased incidence of autoimmune disease and allergy. Also, they may be subject to severe life-threatening anaphylactic reactions to blood products if they have developed a hypersensitivity to the IgA from previous transfusions. In normal concentration, IgA is too diffuse to be seen by HRE. However, in patients with IgA myeloma, or with cirrhosis, which results in a chronically elevated IgA (Chapter 3), a discrete increase in the beta and beta-gamma zone (beta-gamma bridging) is seen respectively.

IgE

Except in the extremely rare case of an IgE myeloma, IgE is insufficient to be seen by HRE. IgE is the immunoglobulin class that is elevated in atopic conditions and in parasitic infestations. In allergies, antigen-specific IgE attaches to mast cells in the mucosa and skin. When the specific allergen attaches to

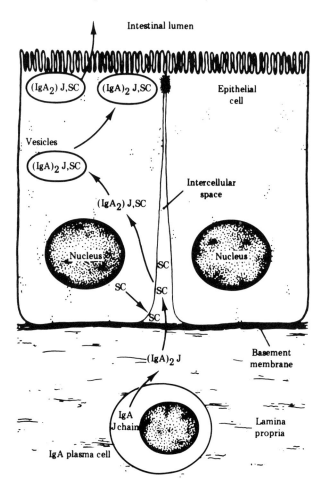

Figure 2-20.   Schematic representation of normal IgA synthesis by plasma cells in the lamina propria. Following synthesis, IgA attaches to the secretory component (an epithelial cell product) and is transported into the intestinal lumen. From reference 56 (used with permission).

these cells, it causes an immediate release of the mast cell products that are responsible for the acute symptoms seen. Recently, it has become clear that reagenic antibodies such as IgE play an important role in host defense against parasitic infections [56].

IgD

Similarly, IgD is not seen by HRE under normal circumstances. While having only a minor defined role in the serum, IgD is one of the major immunoglobulin classes found on the surface membrane of B lymphocytes (Chapter 4). It can be seen by HRE when the patient has an IgD myeloma. One interesting feature of the latter is that whereas most heavy chain classes of myeloma proteins express either kappa or lambda in a normal 2:1 ratio, IgD myelomas have an overwhelming predominance of lambda with a kappa/lambda ratio of 1:9.

Other Gamma Bands

Lastly, numerous small bands can be found in the gamma region of HRE strips. Some of these reflect circulating immune complexes. Kelly et al. [57] pointed out that circulating immune complexes will often appear as two parallel bands in the gamma region. When we see such bands (Figure 2–21), we note that they are present and that this is a pattern that can be seen with circulating immune complexes. Other processes also result in the production of small gamma region bands. This has caused concern and confusion in the past, because with the five-band resolution electrophoretic patterns one could not distinguish a band produced by a monoclonal proliferation of plasma cells until it was sizable and of obvious clinical significance.

With HRE, one can recognize much smaller bands that may be due to

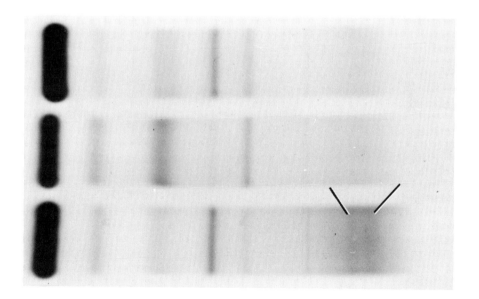

Figure 2–21. Bottom sample shows the parallel lines in the gamma region (*indicated*) that have been associated with circulating immune complexes. Note that similar lines can be seen in patients with monoclonal gammopathies and oligoclonal expansions. They should be interpreted in the particular context for each patient. In patients with hepatitis, such complexes are often seen in the slow gamma region in the context of a polyclonal increase in globulins.

a variety of benign and malignant processes (Chapter 3). The additional information from the HRE patterns does require interpretation and often direct communication with the clinician to determine the relevance of these findings to the individual case. Such communication concerning laboratory findings is not unique for HRE pattern interpretation or even for clinical pathology. Proper interpretation of endometrial samples requires information about age and day of cycle; proper interpretation of upper gastrointestinal tract biopsies requires that the site of biopsy be specified. The additional information provided by HRE can be extremely valuable for determining the diagnosis in a particular case. But if the laboratorian tries to work in isolation without contacting the clinician about problem cases, the interpretations rendered will often be irrelevant to the clinical situation and may mislead the clinician. As with most situations requiring expertise, the laboratorian must recognize his or her limitations and use rather than ignore the additional information in the context of the particular patient's symptomatology.

REFERENCES

1. Westermark P, Pitkanen P, Benson L, Vahlquist A, Olofsson BO, Cornwell III GG. Serum prealbumin and retinol-binding protein in the prealbumin-related senile and familial forms of systemic amyloidosis. Lab Invest 1985;52:314-318.
2. Laurell DB. Composition and variation of the gel electrophoretic fractions of plasma, cerebrospinal fluid and urine. Scand J Clin Lab Invest 1972;29; [Suppl] 124:71-82.
3. Daniels JC. Carrier protein abnormalities. In: Ritzmann SE, Daniels JC, eds. Serum protein abnormalities, diagnostic and clinical aspects. Boston: Little, Brown, 1975:213-242.
4. Bennhold H, Kallee E. Comparative studies on the half-life of 131I-labeled albumins and nonradioactive human serum albumin in a case of analbuminemia. J Clin Invest 1959;38:863-872.
5. Bennhold H, Dlaus D, Schlurlen PG. Volume regulation and renal function in analbuminemia. Lancet 1960;ii:1169-1170.
6. Platt HS, Barron N, Giles AF, Midgley JEM, Wilkins TA. Thyroid-function indices in an analbuminemic subject being treated with thyroxin for hypothyroidism. Clin Chem 1985;31:341-342.
7. Lessard F, Bannon P, Lepage R, Joly JG. Light chain disease and massive proteinuria. Clin Chem 1985;31:475-477.
8. Sunderman Jr FW. Recent advances in clinical interpretation of electrophoretic fractionations of the serum proteins. In: Sunderman FW, Sunderman Jr FW, eds. Serum proteins and the dysproteinemias. Philadelphia: J.B. Lippincott, 1964: 323-345.
9. Fredrickson DS. The inheritance of high density lipoprotein deficiency (Tangier disease). J Clin Invest 1964;43:228-236.
10. Janik B. High resolution electrophoresis and immunofixation of serum proteins on cellulosic media. Ann Arbor: Gelman Sciences;1985:4.

11. Morse JO. Alpha-1 antitrypsin deficiency. N Engl J Med 1978;229:1045–1048.
12. Sharp HL. The current status of alpha-1 antitrypsin, a protease inhibitor in gastrointestinal disease. Gastroenterology 1976;70:611–621.
13. Erikkson S. Studies on alpha-1 antitrypsin deficiency. Acta Med Scan [Suppl] 1965;432:6–12.
14. Keren DF, DiSante AC, Bordine SL. Densitometric scanning of high resolution electrophoresis of serum: methodology and clinical application. Am J Clin Pathol 1986; 85:348–352.
15. Malfait R, Gorus F, Sevens C. Electrophoresis of serum protein to detect alpha-1 antitrypsin deficiency: five illustrative cases. Clin Chem 1985;31:1397–1399.
16. Mullins RE, Miller RL, Hunter RL, Bennett B. Standardized automated assay for functional alpha-1 antitrypsin. Clin Chem 1984;30:1857–1860.
17. Berninger RW, Teixeira MF. Alpha-1 antitrypsin: the effect of anticoagulants on the trypsin inhibitory capacity, concentration and phenotype. J Clin Chem Clin Biochem 1985;23:277–281.
18. Qizilbash A, Young-Pong O. Alpha-1 antitrypsin liver disease differential diagnosis of PAS-positive, diastase-resistant globules in liver cells. Am J Clin Pathol 1983;79:697–702.
19. Eriksson S, Larsson C. Purification and partial characterization of PAS-positive inclusion bodies from the liver in alpha-1 antitrypsin deficiency. N Engl J Med 1975;292:176–180.
20. Larsson C, Kirdsen H, Sundstrom G. Lung function studies in asymptomatic individuals with moderately (PiSZ) and severely (PiZ) reduced levels of alpha-1 antitrypsin. Scand J Respir Dis 1976;57:267–280.
21. Hutchison DGS, Tobin MJ, Cook PJL. Alpha-1 antitrypsin deficiency: clinical and physiological features in heterozygotes of Pi type SZ. Br J Dis Chest 1983;77:28–34.
22. Pierce JA, Eradio B, Dew TA. Antitrypsin phenotypes in St. Louis. JAMA 1975;231:609–612.
23. Morse JO, Lebowitz MD, Knudson RJ. Relation of protease inhibitor phenotypes to obstructive lung disease in a community. N Engl J Med 1977; 296:1190–1194.
24. Stjernberg N, Beckman G, Beckman L, Nystrom L, Rosenhall L. Alpha-1 antitrypsin types and pulmonary disease among employees at a sulphite pulp factory in northern Sweden. Hum Hered 1984;34:337–342.
25. Buffone GJ, Stennis BJ, Schimbor CM. Isoelectric focusing in agarose: classification of genetic variants of alpha-1 antitrypsin. Clin Chem 1983;29:328–331.
26. Sveger T. Liver disease in alpha-1 antitrypsin deficiency detected by screening of 200,000 infants. N Engl J Med 1976;294:1316–1321.
27. Jeppson JO, Laurell BB, Franzen B. Alper CA, Forman DT, Tucker ES, Kruse L. Agarose gel electrophoresis. Clin Chem 1979;25:629–638.
28. Henriksen JJO, Petersen MU, Pedersen FB. Serum alpha-1 acid glycoprotein (orosomucoid) in uremic patients on hemodialysis. Nephron 1982;31:24–25.
29. Docci D, Turci F. Serum alpha-1 acid glycoprotein levels in uremic patients on hemodialysis. Nephron 1983;33:72–73.
30. Lee SK, Thibeault DW, Heiner DC. Alpha-1 antitrypsin and alpha-1 acid glycoprotein levels in the cord blood and amniotic fluid of infants with respiratory distress syndrome. Pediatr Res 1978;12:775–777.
31. Philip AGS, Hewitt JR. Alpha-1 acid glycoprotein in the neonate with and without infection. Biol Neonate 1983;48:118–124.

32. Bienvenu J, Lahet C, Divry P, Cotte J, Bethenod M. Serum orosomucoid concentration in newborn infants. Eur J Pediatr 1981;136:181–186.
33. Salier JP, Sesboue R, Hochstrasser K, Schonberger O, Martin JP. Isolation and characterization of an inter-alpha-trypsin inhibitor-IgG complex from human serum. Biochim Biophys Acta 1983;742:206–214.
34. Papiha SS, Bernal JE, Mehrotra M. Genetic polymorphism of serum proteins and levels of immunoglobulin and complements in high caste community (Brahmins) of Madhya Pradesh India. Jpn J Hum Genet 1980;25:1–8.
35. Garber RA, Delapointe L, Morris JW. PGM1 and Gc subtype gene frequencies in a California Hispanic population. Am J Hum Genet 1983;35:773–776.
36. Lee WM, Emerson DL, Werner PAM, Arnaud P, Goldschmidt-Clermont P, Galbraith RM. Decreased serum group-specific component protein levels and complexes with actin in fulminant hepatic necrosis. Hepatology 1985;5:271–275.
37. Petrini M, Galbraith RM, Emerson DL, Nel AE, Arnaud P. Structural studies of T-lymphocyte Fc receptors. J Biol Chem 1985;260:1804–1810.
38. Emerson DL, Arnaud P, Galbraith RM. Evidence of increased Gc:actin complexes in pregnant serum: a possible result of trophoblast embolism. Am J Reprod Immunol 1983;4:185–189.
39. Burtin P, Grabar P. Nomenclature and identification of the normal human serum proteins. In: Bier M, ed. Electrophoresis theory, methods and applications. New York and London: Academic Press. 2:110–156.
40. Daniels JC, Larson DL, Abston S, Ritzmann SE. Serum protein profiles in thermal burns. II. Protease inhibitors, complement factors, and C-reactive protein. J Trauma 1974;14:153–162.
41. Bevilacqua MP, Amrani D, Mossesson MW, Bianco C. Receptors for cold-insoluble globulin (plasma fibronectin) on human monocytes. J Exp Med 1981;153:42–44.
42. Ahmed AG, Klopper A. A method for the separate measurement of the beta- and alpha-components of SP1 in pregnancy serum. Arch Gynecol 1982;231:307–313.
43. Nerenberg ST. Electrophoretic screening procedures. Philadelphia: Lea and Febiger, 1973.
44. Sutton E. The haptoglobins. In: Steinberg AG, Bearn AG, eds. Conference on genetic disease control, 1st, Washington, D.C. New York and London: Grune & Stratton, 1970;VII:163–216.
45. Whicher JT. The interpretation of electrophoresis. Br J Hosp Med 1980;October:348–360.
46. Ritzmann SE, Daniels JC. Serum electrophoresis and total serum proteins. In: Ritzmann SE, Daniels JC, eds. Serum protein abnormalities: diagnostic and clinical aspects. New York: Alan R. Liss, 1982;2:3–26.
47. Wieme RJ. Agar electrophoresis. Amsterdam: Elsevier, 1965.
48. Schultze HE, Heimburger N, Keide K, Haupt H, Storkio K, Schwick HG. Preparation and characterization of alpha-1 trypsin inhibitor and alpha-2 plasmin inhibitor of human serum. In: Proc 9th Congr Eur Soc Haematology. Basel: Karger, 1963:1315–1320.
49. Karlinsky JB, Snider GL, Franzblau C, Stone PJ, Hoppin FG. In vitro effects of elastase and collagenase on mechanical properties of hamster lungs. Am Rev Respir Dis 1976;113:769–777.
50. Heimburger N. Proteinase inhibitors of human plasma—their properties and control functions. In: Reich E, Rifkin DB, Shaw E, eds. Proteases and biological

control. Cold Spring Harbor Conf Cell Proliferation. Cold Spring Harbor Laboratory, 1975;2:367–386.

51.   Brissenden JE, Cox DW. Alpha-2 macroglobulin in patients with obstructive lung disease, with and without alpha-1 antitrypsin deficiency. Clin Chim Acta 1983;128:241–248.

52.   Klein J. Complement and other activation systems. In: Klein J, ed. Immunology, the science of self-nonself discrimination. New York: Wiley, 1982:310–347.

53.   Pepys MB. C-reactive protein fifty years on. Lancet 1981; i:653–657.

54.   Ramos CE, Tapia RH. C-reactive protein. Lab Med 1984;15:737–739.

55.   Nisonoff A. Introduction to molecular immunology. 2nd ed. Sunderland, MA: Sinauer, 1984.

56.   Keren DF. Immunology and immunopathology of the gastrointestinal tract. Chicago: American Society of Clinical Pathology Press, 1980.

57.   Kelly RH, Scholl MA, Harvey VS, Deveny AG. Qualitative testing for circulating immune complexes by use of zone electrophoresis on agarose. Clin Chem 1980;26:396–402.

CHAPTER 3

Interpretation of High-Resolution Electrophoresis Patterns in Serum, Urine, and Cerebrospinal Fluid

APPROACH TO PATTERN INTERPRETATION

1. Use all the information available to you—both clinical and laboratory.
2. Use a consistent logical approach.
3. Know the basics: Chapter 2.
4. Know the artifacts: application problems, desiccation, hemolysis, incomplete clotting, and improperly labeled specimens.
5. Use a densitometric scan as adjunctive information.
6. When you have found a pattern you do not understand, call the clinician for more information.

As with any clinical laboratory method, one must use a control serum on each electrophoretic strip. We recommend using one at each end of the gel. Commercially available lyophilized control serum and cerebrospinal fluid specimens are convenient and have worked well in our hands to assure adequate migration of the sample. One should be aware of problems with such controls. For example, C3 is usually cleaved into C3c, altering the beta region (Figure 3–1); densitometric scanning of control serum provides objective criteria to determine whether the percentage in the major bands is within an acceptable range. Although some laboratories interpret high-resolution electrophoresis (HRE) strips without densitometric scanning, the information available from densitometry is useful in quality control, confirming impressions from direct visual examination of the HRE strip and following patients with monoclonal gammopathies.

Many earlier authors associated subtle pattern changes with specific conditions. Whereas it is possible to make specific diagnoses from the HRE patterns, overreading minor alterations can result in a loss of confidence by the clinician. For instance, while it is true that minor elevations of the alpha-2

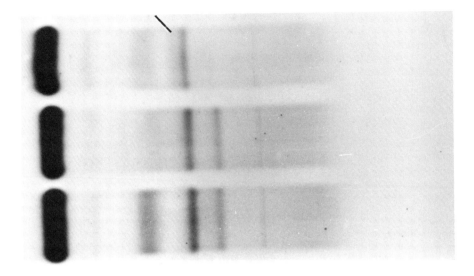

Figure 3-1.   Top sample is from lyophilized control serum. The C3c band is indicated; the normal C3 band is absent.

globulin region often may be seen in patients with malignancies and chronic infections, this is far too nonspecific a finding to include in an interpretive report.

Initial Processing of the Sample

When the patient's sample is received in the laboratory with a request for serum protein electrophoresis, we check the laboratory file for any previous immunoelectrophoretic studies performed on this patient and provide these files with the present material to the pathologist at the time of sign-out. We strongly recommend that clinicians provide us with pertinent information on the requisition slip. Sign-out of the electrophoretic patterns is scheduled daily in midafternoon to coincide with completion of all electrophoretic and specific protein quantitative studies. In addition to the immunology laboratory files, the laboratory computer system provides us with immediate access to all previous studies performed on that patient by all the clinical laboratories in our institution.

Overview of the Electrophoretic Strip

The electrophoretic strip is first examined for the overall electrophoretic migration and staining of the bands. With a control serum at the top and bottom of each strip, one can quickly determine whether there has been any major problem with the gel. Such problems are unusual, but an obvious gel defect is shown in Figure 3-2. A review of the densitometric values for the control serum also provides reliability for these values for the patient samples of that run.

A consistent approach in examining HRE strips must be used to avoid missing significant, although sometimes subtle, alterations. Migration should be consistent from one sample to the next. By reading down the strip, the examiner can use adjacent samples as visual controls. One can easily note decreases in concentration or subtle anodal slurring of albumin caused by drug or bilirubin binding. After reviewing albumin, we proceed cathodally, observing the alpha-1 region for increase or decrease in concentration and alteration of electrophoretic mobility of the alpha-1 antitrypsin band. A common error is overlooking a double alpha-1 band or a shift in the band. This error is usually due to reading across each patient's sample individually instead of comparing them to adjacent bands.

In the alpha-2 and beta regions, common findings include a shift of haptoglobin as a result of hemolysis and activations of C3 to C3c. These alterations can be easily missed, but are obvious when reading down the strip. More subtle findings such as transferrin variants, beta-migrating monoclonal gam-

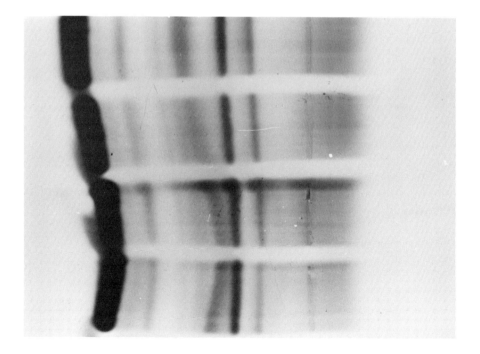

Figure 3-2. Bottom two samples suffer from a gel distortion. Note that both C3 and transferrin bands are straight, indicating that the samples were applied correctly.

mopathies, and minimonoclonal gammopathies can all be seen best by reading down the strip.

INTERPRETATION OF THE INDIVIDUAL PATIENT'S SAMPLE

After the entire strip has been examined and abnormalities noted, the pattern for each patient is reviewed and compared to the densitometric scan. When an abnormality such as an increase in the alpha-1 region is suggested by the initial review, it is useful to have objective, quantitative corroboration by the densitometric scan. However, we rely more on the visual inspection of the gels than the densitometric measurements, because the eye is more sensitive to subtle alterations in migration and staining intensity than is the densitometer instrumentation presently available. This may well change in the future; even today with newer densitometers one can alter the gain and pick up tiny band shifts barely visualized on inspection of the strip (Figure 3–3). Until more sensitive densitometers become standardized, we rely primarily on the visual inspection with densitometry as an adjunctive procedure. It is worth pointing out, however, that more times than I would like to admit a decrease in alpha-1 globulin or gamma globulin was detected only after reviewing the densitometer information. In these cases, the densitometer is acting as a backup to prevent underreading of the gels.

When the electrophoretic strip, densitometer information, appended clinical information, and our laboratory file data on that sample have been reviewed, an interpretation is written for each sample. We have developed coded phrases for many commonly observed patterns and have entered these into the laboratory computer (Table 3–1). We reserve the ability to write a narrative report, when necessary.

In some cases, interpretation cannot be completed until the clinician has been contacted. As emphasized throughout this volume, we are quick to contact clinicians for a variety of reasons: when we observe a significant abnormality not mentioned by the clinician in the history, when we have a pattern that is unusual and does not fit into a typical disease pattern, or when there has been a change in the pattern from a previous HRE sample. We also contact the clinician to cancel needless repetitions of HRE (often, too many house officers order tests on a patient, or there is a misunderstanding of what can be learned from serial HRE studies). Canceling of such needless tests has always been good laboratory practice, but as the laboratory is now viewed as a cost center, this is an absolute necessity for cost-efficient management.

Serum Pattern Diagnosis

Why bother learning pattern diagnosis for HRE? Usually, this is not the most specific way to make a diagnosis. However, pattern recognition is an excellent

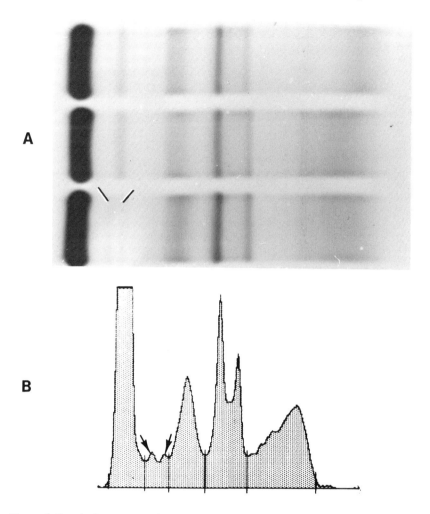

Figure 3-3. A. Lower sample shows two faintly stained bands in the alpha-1 region (*indicated*) compared to the normal alpha-1 regions in the two other samples. B. A densitometric scan in which the alpha-1 region abnormalities (*arrows*) can be seen by enhancing the sensitivity.

screening technique for a wide variety of abnormalities which is useful in suggesting or confirming a clinical diagnosis. There are analogies to tissue pathology pattern recognition; for example, a collection of chronic inflammatory cells may suggest the diagnosis of tuberculosis, fungal infection, autoimmune disease, or lymphoma. To complete the diagnosis, it is necessary to correlate the pattern and clinical information with additional testing such as acid-fast stains, fungal stains, autoantibody testing, or lymphocyte surface marker assays. Similarly, the finding of an unusual HRE pattern suggesting elevated

Table 3–1   Coded Phrases for Common High-Resolution Electrophoresis Patterns on Serum

---

Normal serum protein electrophoresis
Normal IgG, IgA, and IgM levels
Normal kappa/lambda ratio
Immunofixation does not seem to be indicated
Immunofixation is pending
Slightly decreased gamma globulin
Hypogammaglobulinemia
Recommend urine IEP if light chain disease is part of the differential diagnosis
Polyclonal increase in gamma fraction
Increase in ____ IgG, ____ IgA, ____ IgM
Recommend quantification of serum immunoglobulin
Monoclonal spike is present. Rule out myeloma
Small restriction in gamma region; recommend immunofixation of serum and IEP
  of urine
Recommend follow-up in ____ months
Gamma spike persists ([type])
Previously known ____ monoclonal gammopathy
Immunofixation is not indicated
"Tented" restriction in midgamma region suggests the presence of circulating
  immune complexes
Elevated alpha-1 and alpha-2 globulin, consistent with acute phase pattern
Nephrotic pattern
Low albumin
Liver disease cirrhosis pattern
Liver disease hepatitis pattern
Other _____

Note: Includes relevant nephelometric information.

steroid hormone levels should be followed up by specific assays to establish the cause, which may range from birth control pills or pregnancy to a steroid hormone-producing neoplasm. As always, understanding the clinical situation is critical to providing a useful interpretation. For instance, including "birth control pill effect" or "pregnancy pattern" as part of the interpretation of the HRE pattern for a middle-aged man (whose age and sex were not provided, but which you didn't bother to determine) may be a good source of humor on the clinical ward, but will do little to enhance the laboratory's credibility.

Liver Disease Patterns

Cirrhosis

The electrophoretic changes that occur with advanced cirrhosis were among the earliest of the clinically relevant patterns described [1]. The pattern consists of hypoalbuminemia, elevated alpha-1 antitrypsin, polyclonal hypergamma-globulinemia, beta–gamma bridging, and often, decreased haptoglobin [2] (Figure 3–4).

This relatively complex pattern is the result of several pathophysiological alterations. Synthesis of albumin and other proteins is affected by the number of hepatocytes, their current state of health (damage by ethanol, toxins, or biologic agents), and the nutritional and metabolic status of the individual resulting from diet and hormonal changes [3]. Clearly, when sufficient hepatocytes are damaged, synthesis of albumin will be decreased, but this is not necessarily the cause of hypoalbuminemia in most cases of cirrhosis.

Although considerable loss of hepatocytes has occurred in patients with cirrhosis and ascites, the overpowering reserve capacity of the liver can result in a normal or even elevated synthesis of serum albumin in some of these individuals [4]. Therefore, hypoalbuminemia in many individuals relates to the altered distribution of albumin resulting from ascites. Attempts to remove the ascites result in an absolute loss of albumin.

The degree of hypoalbuminemia is too complex to be directly translated into prognosis [5]. When hyperbilirubinemia accompanies the liver disease, the bilirubin binds to albumin, causing an anodal slurring of this band (Figure 3–4). In addition to albumin, other hepatocyte-derived proteins including alpha-1 acid glycoprotein (orosomucoid) and haptoglobin are usually decreased [2]. Whereas prealbumin is decreased consistently and serves as a sensitive

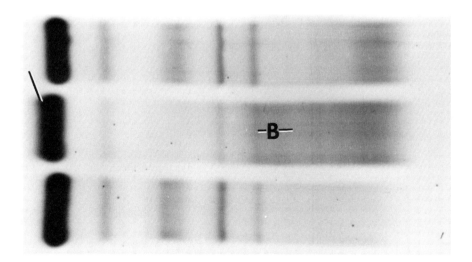

Figure 3–4.   Center serum has a classic cirrhosis pattern. Albumin is slightly decreased and moved anodally (*indicated*) due to bilirubin binding. The alpha-2 region is quite low. Prominent beta–gamma bridging (–B–) is seen together with a polyclonal increase in gamma globulin. Note that top sample has a diffuse increase in the slow gamma region.

indicator of the level of hepatocyte function [6], detection of this is not reliable when using diluted serum for HRE, as in our laboratory method. Undiluted serum might offer a better glimpse at the prealbumin by HRE, but one would pay the price of higher background staining with obscuring of the more important monoclonal bands.

Although transferrin is often decreased in cirrhosis, this is difficult to detect on HRE because of the increased IgA, which has a beta migration and obscures the beta region. Indeed, the beta–gamma bridging relates to a marked elevation in the level of IgA. Normally, the Kupffer cells in the liver remove antigenic material absorbed from the gastrointestinal tract and function to inhibit the immune response to these enteric antigens. In cirrhosis, the portal venous circulation largely bypasses the liver and thereby reaches the systemic immune system. Experimental studies have shown that the increased serum IgA seen in cirrhotic patients can be mimicked by altering the blood flow via a portocaval shunt [7]. The preferential production of IgA may relate to the presence of specific T lymphocytes that augment the IgA response to enterically presented antigens. There is also considerable increase in the IgM and IgG levels, which complete the "bridge" and are responsible for the polyclonal increase in gamma globulin. As further evidence that the increased gamma globulin relates to enteric antigen, it has been shown that the peripheral blood B lymphocytes of patients with cirrhosis have a considerably greater ability to produce IgG to colonic flora than do B lymphocytes from control individuals [8]. In addition, patients with accompanying cholestasis have elevated secretory IgA levels in serum [9].

The other major proteins that increase in cirrhosis are alpha-1 antitrypsin and alpha-2 macroglobulin. Both may be functioning to inhibit proteases released during the ongoing tissue damage in many of these patients. As the increase usually accompanies hypoalbuminemia, some have suggested that alpha-2 macroglobulin may serve to restore the oncotic pressure [10]. The latter seems unlikely, as the increased immunoglobulins more than make up the difference in most cases. Another possibility is that the alpha-2 macroglobulins may be increased as the result of the hyperestrogenic effect seen in many of these patients.

The lipoproteins can confuse the HRE patterns of patients with cirrhosis, as alpha-1 lipoproteins (HDL) are usually decreased while beta lipoproteins (LDL) are increased during biliary obstruction with jaundice [2,11].

Hepatitis

During active hepatic injury, relevant changes of the HRE pattern occur prior to the development of cirrhosis. However, these are too nonspecific to be interpreted as such without supportive clinical and/or laboratory information.

Although considerable ongoing injury results from inflammation, the concentrations of most of the proteins associated with an acute inflammatory reaction pattern (discussed later) are in the normal range. Specifically, alpha-

1 acid glycoprotein (orosomucoid), alpha-1 antichymotrypsin, and C-reactive protein are usually in the normal range while haptoglobin is either normal or reduced. Transferrin, which is usually decreased in the acute inflammatory reaction pattern, is in the normal or elevated range in most of these patients. Only alpha-1 antitrypsin follows the usual acute reaction pattern by being elevated in patients with active hepatic injury [12]. Obviously, some exceptions to these findings occur such as occasional elevations of C-reactive protein (especially early in the disease).

Most patients with hepatitis have normal serum albumin levels. However, an anodal slurring resulting from attachment of their elevated bilirubin is often seen on the albumin band (Figure 3-5). As in cirrhosis, the alpha lipoproteins are usually decreased, but the beta lipoproteins show no reliable changes during hepatitis.

Examination of the gamma globulin region can supply useful information about hepatitis patients. A polyclonal gammopathy, occasionally with oligoclonal bands or parallel bands indicating the presence of circulating immune complexes (see later discussion), is usually seen during clinically active hepatitis (Figure 3-5). A decrease of the polyclonal gammopathy is usually associated with an improving clinical picture [13].

Patients with acute hepatitis usually have a polyclonal gammopathy initially that may become more pronounced if the disease progresses but usually

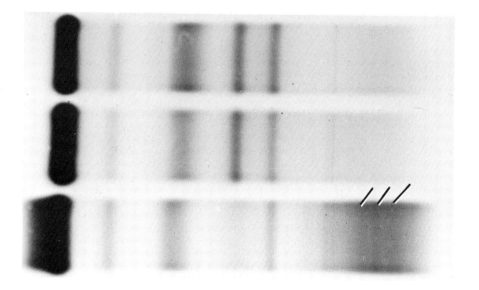

Figure 3-5. Bottom sample is from patient with hepatitis. The anodal slurring is caused by bilirubin binding and is similar to that of Figure 3-4. In the slow gamma region, several prominent bands (*indicated*) are superimposed on a polyclonal (diffuse) increase in gamma globulin. There is no beta–gamma bridging.

regresses with clinical improvement. Frequently, areas of restricted mobility in the slow gamma region may be mistaken for monoclonal gammopathies [14]. The interpreter should be wary of the detection of a monoclonal protein over the background of a polyclonal pattern. Frequently, the polyclonal expansion will have two, three, or more small discrete bands that reflect an oligoclonal gammopathy. These bands merely reflect the greater expansion of those particular B-cell clones and are more evidence of the polyclonal nature of the process. If immunofixation is performed on such a sample (see later), both kappa and lambda bands usually will be identifed. The polyclonal gammopathy is partially in response to the inciting agent (hepatitis A, B, or non-A, non-B) and also due to a similar mechanism as described under cirrhosis. Since the vascular flow through the liver is impeded by the swollen hepatocytes, the same shunting of intestinally derived antigens to the peripheral tissues will occur as in cirrhosis. The better prognosis, found in individuals whose polyclonal gammopathy regresses, reflects recovery of normal hepatocyte structure with restoration of more normal intrahepatic blood flow.

Biliary Obstruction

Biliary obstruction is an end result of a wide variety of disease processes, which may involve the hepatic parenchyma proper, such as in primary bilary cirrhosis, or may result from external obstruction of the biliary tree by stones, inflammation, or neoplasm. The main effect on the HRE pattern results from the elevated bilirubin, which binds to albumin and results in its anodal slurring. Additional irregularities may include acute phase reaction, elevated C3, lipoprotein abnormalities, or an elevated gamma globulin, especially in patients with primary biliary cirrhosis. The latter usually have an elevated IgM level, and circulating immune complexes are common (see later). Nothing about these patterns in themselves allows a specific diagnosis. Albumin is normal or only slightly decreased in concentration and IgA is only slightly elevated (therefore, no beta–gamma bridge is seen), which is helpful in the differential diagnosis from the cirrhosis and hepatitis patterns.

Renal Disease Pattern

When renal disease is severe enough to produce the nephrotic syndrome, HRE demonstrates a characteristic pattern consisting of a low serum albumin, occasionally with anodal slurring, decreased or low normal alpha-1 globulin, and decreased gamma globulin. The alpha-2 region and the beta regions are often elevated (Figure 3–6).

    The nephrotic pattern is the end result of loss of serum proteins through the damaged nephron and the body's attempts to restore the oncotic pressure by overproduction of large proteins that do not pass through the damaged

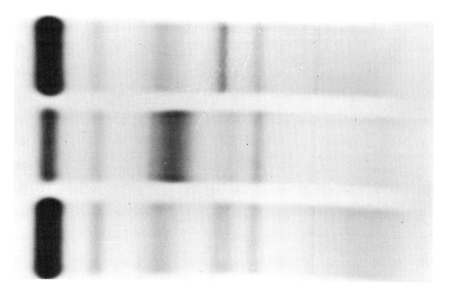

Figure 3-6. Middle sample is typical for a nephrotic pattern. Both albumin and gamma globulin are low; there is a prominent increase in the alpha-2 region. Note that the bottom sample is from a patient with a transferrin variant. Two distinct bands can be seen.

glomeruli. Nephrotic syndrome is defined as proteinuria(>3 g/24 hours), hypoproteinemia, edema, and hyperlipidemia. HRE of serum will only detect the severe cases of renal damage and is of little help in defining the specific site of damage in the nephron. However, examination of the urine by routine urinalysis together with HRE of the urine (discussed later) can help to determine the source of proteinuria. The degree of renal damage will be the main determinant as to abnormality of the serum HRE pattern. Although more than 3g of proteinuria/24hours/1.73 m^2 of body surface area is usually cited as part of the definition of the nephrotic syndrome, it is clear that considerably less proteinuria can produce a clinical picture of nephrosis, especially in children having a relapse of renal disease [15].

Typically, the smaller proteins such as prealbumin, albumin, alpha-1 glycoprotein, alpha-1 antitrypsin, and transferrin are lost into the urine. Depending on the degree of damage, somewhat larger proteins such as IgG may also be lost. The loss of albumin and other proteins into the urine decreases the oncotic pressure, resulting in edema. As a compensatory mechanism, the synthesis of serum proteins is increased. Being larger proteins, alpha-2 macroglobulin and beta lipoprotein (see Chapter 2) do not pass through even moderately damaged glomeruli and are retained in the serum. Indeed, many such patients will have alpha-2 macroglobulin as the major serum protein. For this reason, dye binding analysis by autoanalyzer gives an inaccurate assessment of serum albumin levels in nephrotic patients. Dyes such as bromcresol green will bind to alpha-2 macroglobulin as well as to albumin. While this is a trivial and relatively constant factor in normal serum, it results in a gross overestimation of the serum albumin in nephrotic patients. The serum albumin of the latter individuals should be measured by specific immunoassay (such as nephelometry) or by performing a densitometric scan of HRE of serum (Chapter 2).

Elevated cholesterol in patients with nephrotic syndrome is directly related to the increased beta lipoprotein [16,17]. Due to the self-aggregation that occurs with beta lipoprotein at elevated concentrations (Chapter 2), its electrophoretic mobility is slowed and it appears as an irregular band cathodal to its usual location. Samples from patients receiving hemodialysis may be incompletely clotted due to the heparin that they are given during their therapy. In addition to a band in the fibrinogen region, the heparin will bind to albumin resulting in the anodal slurring described above.

Gastrointestinal Protein Loss

Damage to the gastrointestinal tract will affect the HRE pattern in a variety of ways. Acute damage such as with invasive bacteria or acute exacerbations of inflammatory bowel disease produce an acute phase reaction pattern (Figure 3–7). In addition, depending on the extent and severity of the process, absorption of nutrients including amino acids may be impaired and serum protein may be lost into the lumen of the bowel.

Protein-losing enteropathy may occur at any age as the result of a wide variety of pathologic processes and HRE usually displays hypoalbuminemia, occasionally with decreased gamma globulins. Alpha-2 macroglobulin may be increased as in the nephrotic pattern (Figure 3–8), but in contrast it is unusual to have an elevated beta lipoprotein in patients with protein-losing enteropathies. Whicher [16] has suggested that the amount of protein loss into the gastrointestinal tract can be estimated by measuring the alpha-1 antitrypsin excretion in stool. Obviously, the features of protein-losing enteropathy are far too nonspecific by HRE to suggest a specific diagnosis. However, many patients with disorders such as Whipple's disease do not show clinical symptoms directly referable to the gut until late in the course of their disease [18]. Therefore, the presence of an HRE pattern consistent with protein loss in the bowel is useful information for the clinician. Once again, it should be emphasized that an absolute distinction between a nephrotic and a protein-losing enteropathy pattern cannot be made reliably just from looking at the HRE strip. Clinical history and ancillary laboratory information are significant for the diagnostic process.

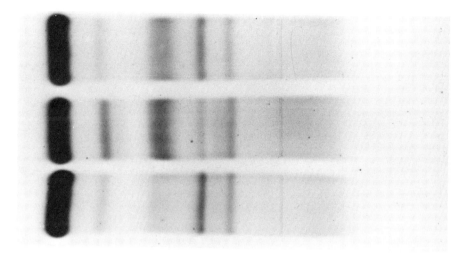

Figure 3-7. Middle sample, from patient with active chronic inflammatory bowel disease, has a complex pattern with several features. The alpha-1 and alpha-2 regions are elevated while transferrin is decreased, which is typical for an acute phase reaction. C3 is also increased. However, the broad increase in the gamma globulin is not usually associated with a pure acute phase pattern and is certainly not diagnostic for this particular condition. However, the interpreter can infer that there is acute activity on some chronic inflammatory process.

Protein Loss through Thermal Injury

Thermal injury to the skin results in a large surface area for loss of serum protein. Elevation of acute phase reactants (alpha-1 antitrypsin, alpha-1 antichymotrypsin, and haptoglobin) with decreased albumin and gamma globulins is often seen. The early thermal injury pattern will differ from the nephrotic and protein-losing enteropathy patterns in that the latter will usually show decreased alpha-1 globulin levels.

Acute Phase Reaction Pattern

During acute episodes of tissue damage with or without inflammation, elevation typically occurs in a group of hepatocyte-derived proteins called the acute phase reactants. In addition, a corresponding decrease, which can be helpful in confirming the pattern, occurs in other proteins. Each acute episode of tissue damage will give a slightly different pattern. However, there is enough similarity that the typical HRE pattern from such individuals contains a slightly

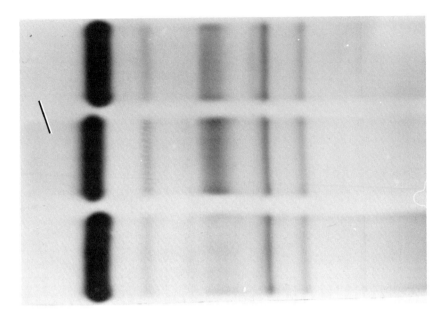

Figure 3-8. Center sample is from patient with protein-losing enteropathy. It is the same as that which would be seen with a mild nephrotic pattern. There is a very faint anodal slurring because the patient was receiving heparin. Albumin was slightly decreased along with the gamma globulin. The alpha-2 region also was increased.

low albumin, elevated alpha-1 globulin with slight anodal slurring, elevated alpha-2 globulin, decreased transferrin, variable C3, and normal or occasionally slightly decreased gamma globulin with a small midgamma band (Figure 3-9).

The time course of an acute phase response following a single episode of tissue injury is outlined in Table 3-2. Initially, the anodal slurring of the alpha-1 band (Figure 3-9) results from the early elevation of alpha-1 acid glycoprotein, which has a more anodal and slightly more diffuse migration than that of alpha-1 antitrypsin (the most common PiM phenotype). C-Reactive protein is usually not detectable by HRE, but with a vigorous acute phase reaction, it may be seen (depending on the electrophoretic system used) as a small band in the midgamma region. As such it may be confused with a small monoclonal gammopathy (see later discussion). By observing the presence of the other elements of the acute phase pattern, and by noting other laboratory values and appropriate clinical history, one will not be led astray. Quantification of the C-reactive protein has been recommended by some studies to detect early infection in patients with leukemia who often do not demonstrate typical granulocyte responses to the infection [19,20].

By 12-24 hours, alpha-1 antitrypsin and haptoglobin levels usually have increased (Table 3-2). The alpha-1 antitrypsin level increases during acute tis-

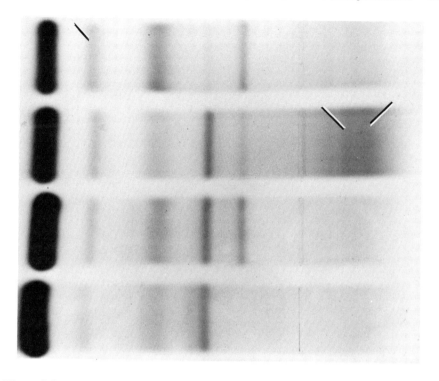

Figure 3–9.   Top serum shows typical uncomplicated acute phase pattern: low albumin, increased alpha-1, and alpha-2, low transferrin. Careful examination (and a little imagination) will disclose the somewhat fuzzy anodal edge of the alpha-1 band, which is due to elevation in the alpha-1 acid glycoprotein (*indicated*). The gamma region of the second sample shows an immune complex pattern (*two indicated bands*) superimposed on a polyclonal increase in gamma globulin.

Table 3–2   Time Course of Acute Phase Reactants[a]

Protein	Earliest Elevation	Peak Elevation (hours)
Alpha-1 acid glycoprotein	6–12 hours	48–72
C-Reactive protein	6–12 hours	48–72
Alpha-1 antitrypsin	24 hours	72–96
Haptoglobin	24 hours	72–96
Fibrinogen	24 hours	72–96
C3	4–7 days	—
Gc globulin	4–7 days	—

Source: Data from Fischer CL, Gill CW. Acute phase proteins. In: Ritzmann SE, Daniels JC, eds. Serum protein abnormalities. Diagnostic and clinical aspects. New York: Alan R. Liss, 1982:331–350.

[a]Following a single acute episode of tissue damage. Note that many diseases have ongoing tissue injury, which results in a more complicated, overlapping elevation of several components.

sue damage even in patients with alpha-1 antitrypsin deficiency. Indeed, if an alpha-1 antitrypsin deficiency is suspected in a patient with ongoing tissue injury or inflammation, a "normal" alpha-1 antitrypsin level could be found by quantifying this protein. It is important in such individuals to perform a concomitant measurement of C-reactive protein or HRE to be certain that the patient does not have evidence of an acute phase pattern, which would obscure the deficiency of alpha-1 antitrypsin. Pregnancy or use of birth control pills is usually accompanied by an elevation of alpha-1 antitrypsin, but these usually produce an elevation in transferrin as well. Haptoglobin is variable in the acute phase reaction. Although it is usually increased at 24 hours after an acute episode of tissue injury, if considerable hemolysis has accompanied the acute tissue injury, then haptoglobin will bind hemoglobin and this product will be removed by the reticuloendothelial system, resulting in a decreased haptoglobin level [20]. Fibrinogen is increased by 24 hours, but one needs to evaluate *plasma* to observe this. Less consistently, elevations in C3, hemopexin, ceruloplasmin, and Gc globulin are seen within a week after acute tissue damage [21,22].

Several proteins consistently decrease in concentration following an episode of acute tissue injury. These "negative" acute phase reactants are useful guides in distinguishing an acute phase pattern from estrogen effect as described above. Typically the albumin and transferrin bands will decrease within a few days following injury. Although prealbumin and alpha lipoprotein also decline, such a decrease would not reliably be detected by HRE.

The acute phase pattern is nonspecific in that it can be seen following a wide variety of tissue injury; however, when some clinical history is provided, its detection can be useful in confirming clinical impressions, in timing an internal injury event, and in predicting infections in patients with impaired leukocyte responses such as individuals with leukemia or others receiving chemotherapy [23]. Further, in patients with known neoplastic conditions, elevated acute phase protein levels have been used as a predictor of tumor necrosis and disseminated disease [24–26]. As stressed previously, the identification of these patterns is not specific. The specimen must be accompanied by a clinical history or the interpreter must contact the clinician to complete the picture for optimal interpretation.

Protein Abnormalities in Autoimmune Disease

While early studies held some promise for the use of electrophoresis in the diagnosis or prognosis of autoimmune diseases [27,28], it has become clear that the findings in these conditions are too nonspecific and varied to provide much useful information. There is often a polyclonal increase in gamma globulin. Further, during active autoimmune disease, circulating immune complexes may produce a limited gamma globulin restricted mobility pattern or an oligoclonal pattern. An acute phase reaction is often seen during acute exacerbations; the alpha-2 may be altered with haptoglobin binding to hemoglobin in episodes of intravascular hemolysis [29]. If a clinical history is provided, the interpreter could comment on the association of the decreased haptoglobin with hemolytic anemia. Overall, screening for autoimmune diseases and, for following particular patients, specific autoantibody titers and evidence of *in vivo* complement activation such as CH_{50} level are more useful than HRE. The intent of this section is to raise the awareness of the interpreter to the variety of patterns that may occur in these patients.

Protein Patterns in Hyperestrogenism

The alterations in hormone balance that occur during pregnancy, in patients taking birth control pills, and in patients with estrogen-producing neoplasms cause changes in many of the serum proteins seen by HRE. During pregnancy, albumin and IgG levels are decreased by 20–25% while alpha-1 antitrypsin and transferrin levels are increased by about 66% (Figure 3–10) [30]. The same

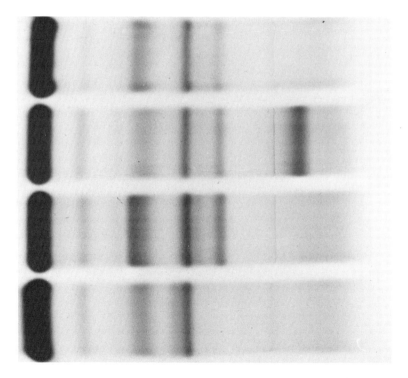

Figure 3–10.   Third sample is from a pregnant young woman. While this is hardly the best way to diagnose pregnancy, it is useful to understand that hyperestrogenism is associated with an elevated alpha-1 lipoprotein (hazy area between albumin and alpha-1 antitrypsin band), along with elevated alpha-1, alpha-2, and transferrin bands. Second sample from top has an obvious monoclonal protein just cathodal to the small origin artifact.

protein alterations are seen in patients taking birth control pills. Since transferrin is not always decreased during acute tissue injury, a proper history will prevent suggesting the presence of an acute phase pattern when the patient is merely taking birth control pills. Moreover, the history of pregnancy with hypertension should alert the reader to pay special notice to the transferrin band, because patients with severe preeclampsia will have a decreased transferrin level [31].

PATTERN INTERPRETATION IN CEREBROSPINAL FLUID

Since the early studies of Kabat et al. [32,33], it has been known that cerebrospinal fluids (CSF) from control individuals have relatively little gamma globulin whereas patients with a variety of neurologic conditions have an elevation of the total CSF protein content with an altered albumin/globulin ratio. In patients with multiple sclerosis and neurosyphilis, there is a considerable increase in the gamma and the prealbumin fractions.

The vast majority of CSF proteins are serum proteins that have passed through the blood–brain barrier at the choroid plexus with only about 20% of CSF proteins synthesized locally [34]. The proteins that pass through the choroid plexus are largely limited by molecular size. Smaller molecules such as prealbumin preferentially pass into the CSF, while larger molecules like alpha-2 macroglobulin and haptoglobin are greatly restricted. This results in a total CSF protein content of only 15–65 mg/dl [35].

To adequately examine the CSF protein bands by HRE, one must either concentrate the sample (we concentrate 80-fold on a commercial ultrafiltration device) and stain with Coomassie blue, or one must use a technique such as silver or immunoperoxidase staining to enhance band visibility. Although there have been several reports of the successful application of silver stains on unconcentrated CSF, the results in our laboratory have been less satisfactory in terms of defining oligoclonal band patterns than on the concentrated samples stained with Coomassie blue. Improvements of silver stain and immunoperoxidase technology will be important areas to watch in increasing both the efficiency and the sensitivity of the laboratory [36,37].

Because of the molecular sieve action of the choroid plexus and the presence of proteins unique to CSF, the HRE pattern of CSF differs considerably from that of serum. Normally, the prealbumin band in serum is barely visible, whereas this band is increased relative to the other protein bands in concentrated CSF (Figure 3–11). Because of the overall bulk of its major protein, the alpha lipoprotein region is weaker than that of the corresponding serum. The alpha-1 antitrypsin band is slightly more diffuse and cathodal in the CSF than in the serum due to desialation of this protease inhibitor within the CSF [16]. As stated previously, the large alpha-2 macroglobulin and haptoglobin molecules do not pass readily into the CSF and therefore the alpha-2 region

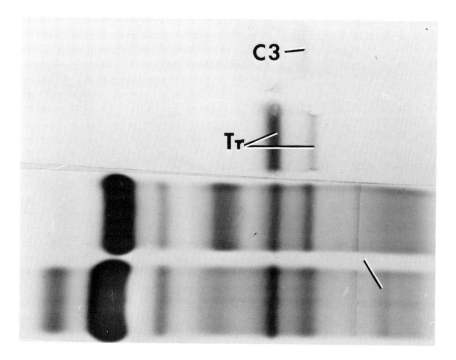

Figure 3–11. Bottom sample is cerebrospinal fluid (CSF) concentrated 80-fold. Immediately above it is a serum sample from the same patient. To demonstrate the makeup of the beta-region bands in the CSF, immunofixation with antitransferrin (Tr) and anti-C3 is shown immediately above. CSF has considerably more prealbumin and considerably less alpha-2 globulin. Also, there is little C3 in CSF; the second beta-region band is composed of desialated transferrin. Note the single band (*indicated*) in the gamma region of CSF; this is often seen and should not be confused with oligoclonal (multiple) bands seen in patients with multiple sclerosis (see Figure 3–12).

is weakly stained in the normal sample. As with serum, the beta region has two major bands; however, unlike serum, the bands reflect different forms of transferrin. The more anodal band (Figure 3–11) is transferrin, which is structurally the same as its serum counterpart. There is relatively little C3 in the CSF, and the second major beta-region band here is mainly a desialated form of transferrin that has been termed the "Tau protein" or "CSF-specific slow transferrin" [38–40]. C3 in the CSF is a weak band just anodal to the desialated transferrin band (Figure 3–11).

As with the serum, the most clinically significant region is the gamma globulin zone. Normally, this region shows little protein even after concentration. The IgG that is present in the CSF tends to show less heterogeneity than serum IgG. In the midgamma region, one can often find a slight sharpening of the gamma band, which may be confused with oligoclonal bands (Figure

3–11) [41,42]. In the slow gamma region, a 10,000-dalton protein called gamma trace protein, which is not an immunoglobulin, is often seen (depending on the method of concentration) [42].

Although there have been several studies of alterations of CSF protein patterns in a wide variety of conditions, including an elaborate classification based on immunoelectrophoresis, there is little clinical diagnostic significance for alterations other than those in the gamma region. Any inflammation involving the meninges results in an elevated CSF total protein due to increased capillary permeability. With increased permeability the total protein content of the CSF increases, as does the proportion of larger proteins such as those in the alpha-2 region. Patients with monoclonal gammopathies will often have this protein present in a small amount within the CSF.

Multiple Sclerosis and Oligoclonal Bands

The most common reason for performing HRE analysis of CSF today is to help in the evaluation of a patient suspected of having multiple sclerosis. It must be emphasized that although the detection of oligoclonal bands in the gamma region is not specific for any disease, examination of the CSF for the presence of oligoclonal bands is helpful because the clinical diagnosis of multiple sclerosis can be difficult and *supportive* laboratory data is useful to the clinician.

Presenting clinical symptoms and signs of multiple sclerosis include weakness, diplopia, optic neuritis, paresthesias and numbness, poor vibration sensation leading to difficulty with coordinated movements, absent abdominal reflexes, trigeminal neuralgia (in young adults), vertigo, and easy fatigability [43]. The diagnosis of multiple sclerosis rests on strict clinically defined features: recurrent episodes of the above phenomena, indicating at least two anatomic sites of involvement. Early on many of these signs and symptoms are nonspecific, and a diagnosis of multiple sclerosis at this stage can be quite difficult. The clinical laboratory has been able to provide some useful information to support the diagnosis in many of these patients.

Two useful tests can be performed by most clinical laboratories. Patients with multiple sclerosis have an increased local (CSF) synthesis of IgG, usually restricted to the antibody products of a few clones (oligoclonal) of B cells and found in the gamma region of the CSF but not in the corresponding serum in over 90% of these patients. Recent evidence has indicated that multiple sclerosis patients lacking oligoclonal bands in the CSF have fewer plasma cells within the meninges and fewer plaques at time of autopsy than patients whose CSF contains oligoclonal bands. This suggested that the oligoclonal bands are a reflection of the local synthesis of immunoglobulin by plasma cells in the diseased tissue [44]. The specific antigen(s) to which these antibodies are being made have not been identified. Patients with multiple sclerosis usually do not have an elevated total CSF protein, as the immunoglobulin synthesized and secreted within the CSF is a relatively small amount compared to the other CSF proteins. As a result of this increased local synthesis of IgG, however, there is a decrease in the albumin/globulin ratio of the CSF that also occurs in other diseases. To correct for decreases in albumin/globulin ratio associated with diseases that merely increase the permeability of the blood–brain barrier, an IgG index is often used [45]:

$$\text{IgG index} = \frac{\text{CSF IgG/serum IgG}}{\text{CSF albumin/serum albumin}}$$

Between 65 and 80% of patients with multiple sclerosis have an elevated IgG index [46]. However, while an elevated IgG index is useful with a patient with the appropriate clinical setting, elevated local production of IgG is also seen in patients with viral encephalitis, bacterial meningitis, neurosyphilis, subacute sclerosing panencephalitis, and Guillain-Barré syndrome [43]. Patients whose CSF IgG elevation is due to the presence of a systemic polyclonal gammopathy with immunoglobulin passively diffusing into the CSF will have a normal IgG index.

With the advent of electrophoretic techniques possessing better resolving power than earlier methods, it became clear that the increased gamma globulin resulted largely from the products of a few clones of plasma cells that gave an oligoclonal pattern by HRE or isoelectric focusing (Figure 3–12) [47]. The local production of immunoglobulin likely has relevance in multiple sclerosis because the production of these clones by particular individuals may be related

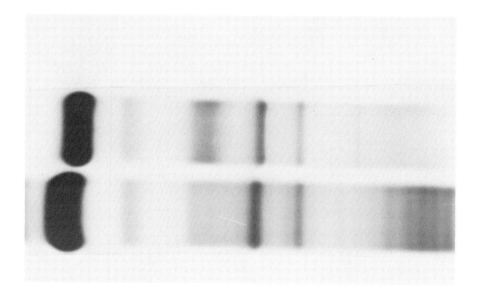

Figure 3–12.   Top sample, serum; bottom, CSF concentrated 80-fold, from patient with multiple sclerosis. Oligoclonal bands are present only in CSF.

to certain inherited capabilities. The evidence for genetic restriction of the disease comes from studies of immunoglobulin subclasses and HLA typing; patients with multiple sclerosis consistently have a restricted response with predominately IgG1 subclass [48]. Further, a linkage of the disease with HLA-A3 and -B7 implies a genetic predisposition to develop this disease [49].

Because IgG is synthesized locally in the central nervous system, the oligoclonal bands in multiple sclerosis patients are present in the CSF and not in the corresponding serum from the same patient [50]. When we find oligoclonal bands in both the CSF and serum, we consider this to be a result of diffusion of the serum oligoclonal bands into the CSF. An occasional case with oligoclonal bands in both locations does occur, but this is not considered useful in confirming the presence of multiple sclerosis; the oligoclonal bands in the serum stain only weakly [46]. The more sensitive isoelectric focusing technique will often find such bands in the serum of patients with multiple sclerosis [51].

Although isoelectric focusing is probably the most sensitive method to detect oligoclonal bands in the CSF, it is not currently being used for routine clinical testing for several reasons. The technique is not yet available in a commercial form that is usable by most clinical laboratories. Unlike HRE, which has its many applications, isoelectric focusing in the routine clinical laboratory is of very limited use, which makes the assay far too costly for the resulting information. Interpretation is difficult due to the large number of bands that are generated and the inexperience of clinical laboratory workers in reviewing such information. Finally, the slightly increased sensitivity has been shown to lead to a greater number of bands in other conditions [46], inadvertently increasing the nonspecificity of the test.

HRE analysis by agarose or by some of the newer acetate methods (Table 3–3) can provide adequate sensitivity while offering broad application in the laboratory and results that are readily interpreted [52]. Authors have recently exhorted the clinical laboratory to be careful of different commercial methods available for performing HRE on CSF [53,54]. We have found that a system

Table 3–3   CSF Oligoclonal Bands by Agarose and Cellular Acute

Diagnosis	Acetate (%)	Agarose (%)
Definite MS[a]	92.8	95.4
Possible MS	38.1	39.8
Not MS	8.0	7.1

Source: Data from Embers GC, and Paty DW. CSF electrophoresis in one thousand patients. Can J Neurol Sci 1980; 7:275–280.
[a]Criteria of multiple sclerosis (MS):
  Definite; clinically definite MS.
  Possible; MS was part of the differential diagnosis.
  Not; MS was not part of the differential diagnosis.

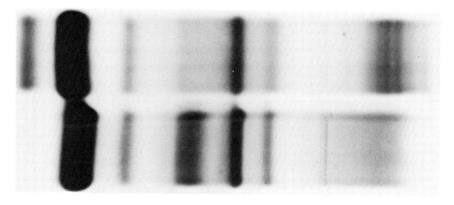

Figure 3-13. Concentrated CSF shows several oligoclonal bands (Panagel system).

with a specific cooling block offers excellent resolution (Figure 3–13). However, other methods with cooling accomplished by convection are available commercially and also produce excellent results (Figure 3–14). Not all systems commercially available have given what our laboratory requires as minimal sensitivity, that is, the ability to detect multiple small bands in patients with multiple sclerosis.

For testing purposes, by mixing a few different monoclonal gammopathies that have different electrophoretic mobilities and then diluting the samples in electrophoresis buffer, the laboratorians can establish a control specimen for comparing different systems. The ultimate test, however, should involve the use of CSF samples run in parallel on both systems. A serum sample from the same patient should always be run adjacent to the concentrated CSF. Although our laboratory will assay CSF samples sent without serum, the report is always appended with "serum should be run with sample to improve

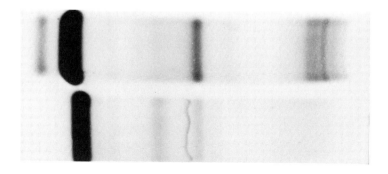

Figure 3-14. Same CSF as in sample in Figure 3–13 shows the same oligoclonal bands (Beckman system).

the specificity of this information.'' We will also accept a serum up to 1 week after the CSF sample was run to assay as the control serum. If the serum had oligoclonal bands, we are confident that in a week they would still be present in a large enough concentration that we would detect them. This cutoff is arbitrary and has not been rigorously investigated.

It is also necessary to define what will be included as an "oligoclonal band pattern." Our laboratory accepts as positive for oligoclonal bands a pattern that has two distinct bands in the gamma region that are not composed of the gamma trace protein band and the slight restriction normally seen with gamma CSF proteins. As with interpretation of serum protein electrophoresis, it is best if the samples can be batched and several assayed at the same time. This will allow the interpreter to compare different samples for the position of gamma trace protein or any other artifactual restriction (Figure 3-11). Further, the counterpart serum, which should be adjacent to the concentrated CSF from the same patient, must not have the same oligoclonal bands. The final interpretation of the specimen depends on the relationship between the CSF and serum patterns. Our laboratory sign-outs are given in Table 3-4.

After going to the trouble to detect oligoclonal bands in the CSF that are not present in the corresponding serum, the laboratorian must realize that the test is not pathognomonic for multiple sclerosis. Indeed, oligoclonal bands can be found in a wide variety of neurologic diseases including inflammation, neoplasia, cerebrovascular accidents, demyelinating diseases, some peripheral neuropathies, and even Whipple's disease (Table 3-5). Except for those patients with subacute sclerosing panencephalitis, the percentage of patients with these conditions having oligoclonal bands is considerably less than that of multiple sclerosis patients, and multiple sclerosis is not part of the differential diagnosis in most of these patients.

Because the test is nonspecific, it should be used in defined situations, such as in the case of a patient who has had only a few clinical episodes suggestive of multiple sclerosis, but the diagnosis is not yet secure. The presence of oligoclonal bands in such patients is useful supportive information. A negative test will cause the clinician to review the clinical features, as 90% of patients with multiple sclerosis should have oligoclonal bands in the CSF. Obviously, the laboratory test should never be used as the sole evidence of multiple sclerosis; some patients with optic neuritis (one early sign that *may* indicate multiple sclerosis) and oligoclonal bands have not developed overt multiple sclerosis after more than a decade of follow-up. Other patients whose CSF lacked oligoclonal bands did develop multiple sclerosis [55,56]. In their study of the predictive values of oligoclonal bands, Gerson et al [57] found that the predictive value of a positive test for oligoclonal bands was 78% and that of a negative test was 89%. Most recent laboratory studies comparing various methods to diagnose multiple sclerosis agree that the best single test is determination of oligoclonal bands in the CSF by agarose gel electrophoresis [57,58]. As with many other interpretations discussed previously, contact with

Table 3-4 Final Interpretation of CSF for Oligoclonal Bands

Situation		Interpretation
CSF	Serum	
Oligoclonal bands present	No oligoclonal bands	CSF is positive for _____ oligoclonal bands
Oligoclonal bands present	Same oligoclonal bands	CSF contains _____ oligoclonal bands. Since the corresponding serum contains the same oligoclonal bands, this is not specific enough to be considered supportive evidence for MS
Oligoclonal bands present	No sample sent	_____ oligoclonal bands are in CSF. Without a corresponding serum sample, we are uncertain as to the significance of these findings. Recommend serum for comparison electrophoresis
One band present	Same band seen	Monoclonal band is present. Recommend kappa/lambda ratio, immunoglobulin quantification, and immunofixation to identity
No oligoclonal bands present	Serum with or without bands	CSF is negative for oligoclonal bands
One band present	No oligoclonal bands	One gamma band is seen. This is insufficient to be supportive evidence for MS

Table 3-5   Conditions in Which Oligoclonal Bands May Be Found in CSF

Multiple sclerosis[a]
Subacute sclerosing panencephalitis
Creutzfeldt-Jakob disease
Meningoencephalitis
Spinal cord compression
Guillain-Barré syndrome
Syphilis
Peripheral neuropathy
Optic neuritis
Hydrocephalus
Cerebrovascular accident
Immune complex vasculitis
Systemic lupus erythematosus
Diabetes
Whipple's disease
Neoplasms
Fever of unknown origin

[a]In multiple sclerosis about 90% of patients will have oligoclonal bands in the CSF. In most of the other conditions listed, such bands are uncommon but *may* be seen.

the clinical services involved helps limit inappropriate use of this test; why do this procedure on a 62-year-old man with an obvious cerebrovascular accident?

Another feature of CSF oligoclonal bands is that the number of bands and their electrophoretic migration tend to remain constant during active and inactive disease over a period of years [59,60]. This is in contrast to myelin basic protein, which is found in the CSF of patients with active but not with inactive multiple sclerosis [61,62].

Optimally, a combination of the IgG index and oligoclonal banding will yield confirmatory evidence in more than 90% of cases with multiple sclerosis. Papadopoulos et al. [63] warned that to minimize errors in laboratory methodology, the same immunochemical method (e.g., nephelometry) should be used to calculate the IgG and the albumin.

Oligoclonal bands in the CSF have also been used for clinical diagnosis in systemic lupus erythematosus (SLE). Some patients with SLE develop central nervous system (CNS) involvement, which can be manifested by a variety of symptoms: psychosis, cranial nerve palsy, seizures, cerebrovascular accidents, and transverse myelopathy [64]. The incidence of CNS manifestations in patients with SLE varies widely from 25%, reported in a large clinical series, to as high as 75% in a retrospective postmortem series [64,65]. It is also clear that CNS involvement can be the cause of death in as many as 13% of these patients [66].

Unfortunately, symptoms of CNS lupus can be mimicked by steroid psychosis, and the clinician is occasionally faced with a patient with known SLE who is receiving steroid therapy and evidencing psychotic symptoms. Should the steroids be increased (for CNS lupus) or should they be tapered (for steroid psychosis)? Over the years, there have been many attempts at establishing laboratory tests that would help with this differential diagnosis. Largely, they have failed. Levels of C3, C4, anti-DNA, and, more recently, oligoclonal bands in the CNS are at best only partially helpful. The clinical picture remains the gold standard for whether the patient has CNS lupus [67].

The increased IgG levels seen in the CNS of some patients with CNS lupus result primarily from an impaired blood–brain barrier. Although the demonstration of oligoclonal bands in the CSF of these patients is interesting, only a minority of the patients with SLE and CNS symptoms had such bands in recent studies [68]. A negative oligoclonal band test in a patient with clinically suspected CNS lupus will not cause the clinician to withhold therapy. On the other hand, a positive oligoclonal band test provides some confirmatory information but is highly nonspecific. In our laboratory, we recommend use of the CSF oligoclonal band test only as a confirmatory test for patients suspected of having multiple sclerosis.

HRE INTERPRETATION FOR URINE

HRE of urine samples can provide useful information as to the composition of proteinuria and, consequently, the location and degree of damage within the nephron. This is possible because the glomeruli and tubules normally allow only small amounts of certain proteins to pass into the urine.

Several factors influence the composition of proteins in the urine, of which protein size is an obvious factor. In general, molecules smaller than albumin pass through the glomerulus while larger molecules are retained in the blood. *Charge* of the protein, however, is also an important factor. While the polyanion albumin is repelled by the negatively charged glomerular capillary surface, neutral dextran of similar molecular weight will pass into the glomerular filtrate [69]. A third factor that may complicate protein composition of urine is the *hydrostatic pressure* within the systemic circulation. As blood pressure increases, larger molecules are forced through the glomerulus. This results in a glomerular filtrate with a disproportionately large amount of molecules larger than 100,000 daltons.

Under normal circumstances, then, the glomerular filtrate is composed of numerous small molecular weight proteins and polypeptides along with albumin (because of its great concentration in serum, some is able to pass through the glomerulus). The most prominent smaller proteins in the glomerular filtrate include alpha-1 acid glycoprotein (orosomucoid, 40,000 daltons), alpha-1 microglobulin (27,000), beta-2 microglobulin (12,000), gamma trace protein, and retinol binding protein (20,000). These proteins are normally reabsorbed by the renal tubules so that in concentrated normal urine only albumin is usually seen by HRE.

In most urine samples, insufficient protein is present for detection by standard HRE techniques. Consequently, the urine must be concentrated (we recommend at least 100-fold) to allow examination of the various fractions. In concentrating the urine, one must be concerned with the possible loss of low molecular weight proteins that are useful to determine the location of damage within the nephron. Commercial concentrators which can be used allow concentration of proteins with a molecular weight above 10,000. This permits smaller molecules with diagnostic significance, such as monomeric Bence Jones proteins, to be included in the sample.

Normally, individuals excrete about 100 mg of protein daily in the urine. Most of this protein is albumin with some gamma globulin and many small molecular weight proteins. The urine HRE has a different protein band pattern than that of serum. Albumin migrates closer to the anode in the urine than in the serum and there is often an anodal slurring that smears the band toward the positive electrode. This migration of albumin is attributed to the binding of anions to its surface [70]. Little prealbumin or alpha-1 acid glycoprotein (orosomucoid) is present in the normal concentrated urine, although alpha-1 acid glycoprotein is more readily cleared through the glomerulus than in albumin. Alpha-1 antitrypsin is well separated and is seen especially well in patients with glomerular proteinuria. Alpha-1 microglobulin is relatively stabile in urine and is useful as an indicator for renal tubular dysfunction [71].

Alpha-2 macroglobulin and haptoglobin are too large to pass into the urine unless there has been severe damage to the nephron. There are, however, other alpha-2 microglobulins such as retinol-binding protein that are not usually seen in the serum but are usually present in the concentrated urine specimen [72]. These alpha-2 microglobulins are relatively stabile in urine, and have been suggested as good markers for the presence of renal tubular disease [73]. Two other bands that denote smaller molecular weight proteins not seen (readily) in serum are beta-2 microglobulin and gamma trace protein. Note that due to the small molecular weight of the latter the conditions of concentrating are a key factor in its detection. Beta-2 microglobulin migrates between transferrin and C3. Since beta lipoprotein does not occur in this region in urine HRE, it is not confused with beta-2 microglobulin [74]. The detection of this protein is useful for estimating tubular damage; however, its presence is variable due to its poor stability in acid urine with pH < 6.0 [75,76].

Very little gamma globulin is present in normal urine. Many investigators incorrectly assume that light chains are not found except when a Bence Jones proteinuria is present. Plasma cells normally will produce excess portions of free light chains that occur as monomers with a molecular weight of about 22,000 or as dimers with a weight of 44,000. As such, they pass through glomeruli and, when present in sufficient amount, are not completely reabsorbed by the tubules, resulting in a light chain proteinuria. They migrate broadly from the alpha-2 region through the slow beta or fast gamma region. In patients with polyclonal increases in the serum gamma globulins, such as individuals with chronic inflammation or autoimmune disease, there is also an excessive production of free light chains, which the casual observer of immunoelectrophoretic patterns can mistake for monoclonal free light chains (Bence Jones protein) (Figures 3–15 and 3–16).

Proteinuria after Minor Injury

The mere detection of protein in the urine is a highly nonspecific although important finding that may result from a wide variety of insults. By identifying the type of proteins leaking into the urine, the laboratorian provides useful information to the clinician. The concept of "selectivity," developed to help estimate the location and degree of injury to the kidney, refers to the ability of the glomerulus to select only smaller proteins for passage through the glomerular basement membrane; that is, the molecular sieve function of the glomerulus. If very large molecules such as IgG leak through the glomerulus in proportion to smaller molecules such as albumin, then the proteinuria is termed "nonselective"; that is, the glomerulus is not able to discriminate between these two molecules. The greater the glomerular damage, the less selective is the proteinuria. Selectivity index is estimated from the ratio of IgG clearance to that of albumin clearance. Its use has been advocated in children in temperate climates with nephrotic syndrome in whom high selectivity is seen in minimal change disease, although in tropical locations the selectivity index is of limited use [77].

Relatively minor injury has been associated with proteinuria. For instance, vigorous physical exercise has been reported to cause as much as a 100-fold increase in protein in the urine [78]. Patients with febrile nonrenal illnesses often have a concomitant proteinuria [79]. During such episodes, both large and small molecular weight protein bands have been reported, indicating a combined tubular and glomerular proteinuria [80]. The etiology of the pro-

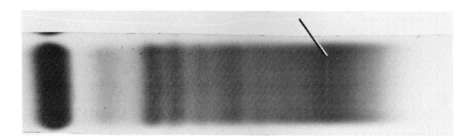

Figure 3–15.   Urine from patient with chronic osteomyelitis. The pattern shows both glomerular and considerable tubular proteinuria. Around the origin, a hazy density (*indicated*) may be confused with Bence Jones protein.

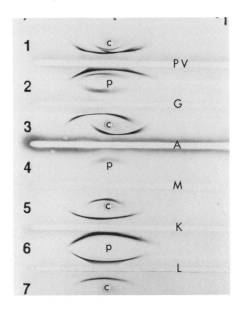

Figure 3-16. Immunoelectrophoresis (IEP) of urine from Figure 3-15 shows a polyclonal increase in light chains. Patient urine (P) alternates with control *serum* (C). Reaction with polyvalent antisera (PV) demonstrated a large arc, which entended into the trough, and two smaller arcs (*indicated*). One small arc reacted with anti-IgG (G) and the other with anti-IgA (A). Typically, there was no reaction with anti-IgM (M). Note that both the antikappa (K) and antilambda (L) precipitin lines extend into the trough, indicating the great concentration of both these light chains. Obviously, unless there is a great amount of IgE or IgD in the urine, most of these light chains are not attached to heavy chains. This is because they are free polyclonal light chains, a relatively common finding often mistaken for Bence Jones protein.

teinuria in these conditions is unclear. While some workers have suggested that it may be related to circulating immune complexes, recent work by Solling et al. [81] indicated that there is no correlation between the presence of circulating immune complexes during nonrenal disease-associated febrile episodes and proteinuria (either glomerular or tubular). Within 2 days after such illness, most of the proteinuria has resolved.

Proteinuria and Renal Disease

More severe renal disease results in a profound proteinuria, the characteristics of which can be defined by HRE in many cases. In general, patients with glomerular disease excrete considerably more protein than those with tubular disease. This reflects the pathophysiology in which tubular dysfunction prevents absorption of the few small proteins that normally pass through the glomerulus, while glomerular disease literally opens the floodgates to large amounts of serum proteins. When glomerular damage occurs, larger molecules pass into the glomerular filtrate along with the same amount of smaller proteins that freely passed into the glomerular filtrate under normal conditions. The smaller proteins and some of the larger molecular weight protein can be reabsorbed by the renal tubules. However, the absorptive capacity is often overwhelmed, and the HRE of the urine reflects the fact that a greater amount of large molecules such as albumin, alpha-1 antitrypsin, and transferrin are present than the smaller molecules [82] (Figure 3–17).

In patients with tubular disease, normal glomerular selectivity is maintained with only small molecules passing into the filtrate. The lack of absorptive capacity by the damaged tubules, however, allows these small proteins to pass into the urine where they are seen upon concentration as small alpha-1, -2, and beta-2 microglobulins (see previous discussion) (Figure 3–18). When looking at these electrophoretic patterns, one sees considerable variation because the amount of nephron damage differs from one to another patient. However, a key feature we use is that albumin is much less dominant and

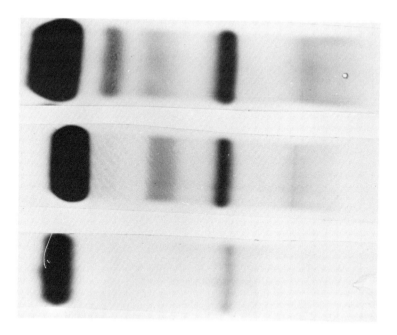

Figure 3–17. Three examples of glomerular proteinuria. Note that the urine samples do not line up exactly because they were electrophoresed on three separate runs. In all three, the main protein excreted is albumin with varying amounts of alpha-1 antitrypsin, transferrin, and other globulins.

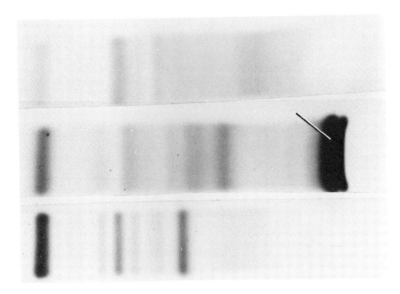

Figure 3-18. Three examples of tubular proteinuria. With tubular proteinuria, the glomeruli are relatively intact and do not allow large amounts of albumin and larger molecules to pass into the glomerular filtrate. Therefore, albumin is relatively minor or at most equivalent to the many smaller molecules seen in the alpha and beta regions. Note that the middle sample is from a patient with kappa Bence Jones protein (*indicated*). The latter sample actually has two fused bands because of the formation of both monomer and dimer kappa chains.

occasionally a relatively minor constituent of tubular proteinuria as compared to glomerular proteinuria. Individuals with more chronic renal disease will often have a combined glomerular and tubular pattern indicative of widespread damage to the nephron (Figure 3-19). In these patients, the albumin content resembles that of glomerular proteinuria, but the smaller bands in the alpha and beta region can also be observed. Therefore, both the amount and type of protein in the urine provide information as to the ongoing disease processes.

Recently, quantification of small molecular weight proteins as an indication of tubular proteinuria has been advocated. The urinary protein most often used to evaluate this is beta-2 microglobulin, a molecule that has homology with immunoglobulins. While it is elevated in tubular proteinuria, it is unstable at $pH < 6.5$ and may result in a false-negative value. Alpha-1 microglobulin is another plasma glycoprotein that passes freely into the urine. It is stable at acid pH and may be a better indicator of tubular dysfunction than beta-2 microglobulin [71]. Other suggested markers for detecting tubular proteinuria include retinol-binding protein, lysozyme, and *N*-acetyl-B-B-glucosaminidase [83].

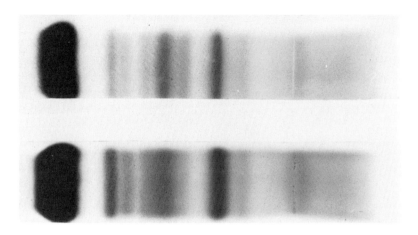

Figure 3-19. Two samples from patients with combined glomerular and tubular proteinuria. Note that while albumin predominates, many discrete bands are present in the alpha and beta regions.

HRE of concentrated urine samples can provide much of this information. In many cases, the tubular or glomerular nature of the process is obvious. When there is considerable proteinuria, the sample may only be concentrated 25-fold or less so as not to overload the gel. Glomerular patterns of injury are usually readily distinguishable from the tubular forms of disease. Unfortunately, HRE does not define the molecular weights of the constituents as does SDS-polyacrilamide gel electrophoresis. However, as the latter technique has considerably less overall use in a clinical laboratory setting, its use is presently quite limited.

Another advantage of performing HRE on urine is that one can detect the presence of monoclonal free light chain (Bence Jones protein). Bence Jones protein was originally defined by its peculiar thermal characteristics; it precipitates when the urine is heated to 40–60°C and redissolves upon boiling. When the urine cools, the protein reprecipitates [84]. In recent years, it has become clear that the protein described was a free light chain from a patient with multiple myeloma. It has also become clear that the old heating test is inadequate by virtue of both nonspecificity and insensitivity. Not all urine with Bence Jones protein (BJP) will behave appropriately upon heating, and polyclonal increases in light chain can give false-positives. Further, patients with glomerular proteinuria with large amounts of transferrin in the urine will give a false-positive heat test for BJP due to the precipitation of transferrin at 60°C and its redissolution at 95°C.

The most sensitive and specific test now for BJP is immunoelectrophoresis. HRE alone will detect most patients with BJP; however, it is too insensitive to detect the small amounts of BJP that occur in some patients, especially some on therapy (Figure 3-20). Immunofixation would be the most sensitive method for detecting BJP; however, in our laboratory we found that for optimal detection, the amount of BJP present needs to be estimated in order to be in the proper dilution for complete immunoprecipitation. As the concentration of the proteins are "automatically" adjusted during the immunoelectrophoresis (IEP) diffusion step, it is the simplest and at present best single test for detecting BJP.

Other workers prefer to use antisera specific for free light chains in a gel diffusion or IEP mode. Unfortunately, commercial antisera specific for free light chains are notoriously heterogeneous in their specificity and in their sensitivity, which a brief word about their mode of production will clarify. First, a purified free light chain is used to immunize a laboratory animal (rabbit or sheep) that will produce antibodies to determinants on the light chain. Most of these antigenic determinants are expressed on the surface of the molecule, whether it is combined with a heavy chain or whether it exists as a free light chain (Figure 3-21). Consequently, these antibodies would form an immunoprecipitate for either free light chains or whole immunoglobulin molecules that contain that light chain. A few determinants are relatively or completely

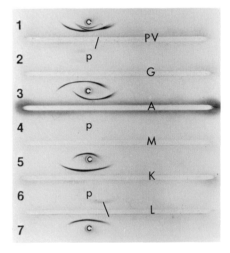

Figure 3-20. Immunoelectrophoresis (IEP) shows a very subtle Bence Jones lambda protein (*indicated*). The protein is seen best reacting with the antilambda (L) reagent, but can be faintly discerned with the antipolyvalent (PV) just cathodal to the weak IgG reaction. Most Bence Jones proteins are obvious on both HRE and IEP of urine. This sample, however, had no protein detected by HRE, and only IEP revealed the subtle lambda Bence Jones protein. This sample is from a patient with known myeloma with previous Bence Jones lambda protein demonstrated. After chemotherapy, there was a marked decrease in the monoclonal protein (present sample). Symbols: p, urine; c, control; K, kappa; A, anti-IgA; G, anti-IgG; M, anti-IgM.

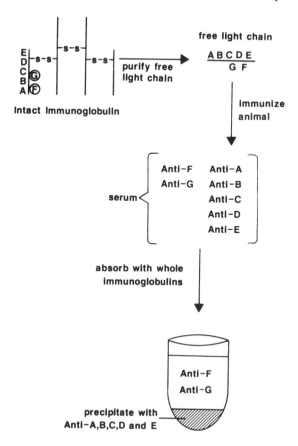

Figure 3–21.   Reactivities to free light chains can be created because some light chain determinants are "hidden" in intact molecules.

hidden when the light chain is combined with the heavy chain. Therefore, the antiserum is absorbed with a large amount of whole immunoglobulin molecules so that the antibodies that react with light chain determinants expressed on an intact molecule will be removed, leaving only those antibodies that react with the determinants that are normally hidden on the intact molecule. The problem with the absorption is that it removes the antibodies heterogeneously and results in a very weak antisera, which may still have a few groups that react weakly with whole molecules.

Additionally, small amounts of free polyclonal light chains can be found in the urine and are increased in a variety of chronic inflammatory conditions. When there is a preponderance of kappa chains, for instance, they could appear as a false-positive, especially if the free lambda chain-specific reagent is relatively weak. Although we have found HRE alone even on 100-fold concentrated urine to be too insensitive to pick up the more subtle cases, most cases of clinically significant BJP can be detected by HRE. Eventually, quantification of kappa and lambda in the urine by nephelometry or some similar technique will provide a better screening test for disproportionate kappa/lambda ratios and will help determine the concentration of specimen that will be run for immunofixation (see subsequent discussion; Chapter 5). Until then, we perform IEP for screening for BJP.

REFERENCES

1. Wuhrman F, Wunderly Ch. Die Bluteiweisskorper des menschen. Basel: Benno Schwabe, Verlag, 1947.
2. Hallen J, Laurell CB. Plasma protein pattern in cirrhosis of the liver. Scand J Clin Lab Invest 1972;29;[Suppl]124:97–103.
3. Rothschild MA, Oratz M, Schreiber SS. Albumin synthesis. N Engl J Med 1972;286:748–753.
4. Rothschild MA, Oratz M, Zimmon D, Schreiber SS, Weiner I, Van Caneghem A. Albumin synthesis in cirrhotic subjects with ascites studied with carbonate. J Clin Invest 1969;48:344–349.
5. Cozzolino G, Francica G, Lonardo A, Cigolari S, Cacciatore L. Lack of correlation between the laboratory findings and a series of steps in the clinical severity of chronic liver disease. La Ricerca Clin Lab 1984;14:641–648.
6. Agostoni A, Marasini B, Stabilini R, Del Ninno E, Pontello M. Multivariate analysis of serum protein assays in chronic hepatitis and postnecrotic cirrhosis. Clin Chem 1974;20:428–429.
7. Thomas HC, McSween RNM, White RG. Role of the liver in controlling the immunogenicity of commensal bacteria in the gut. Lancet 1973;i:1288–1291.
8. Mutchnick MG, Keren DF. In vitro synthesis of antibody to specific bacterial lipopolysaccharide by peripheral blood mononuclear cells from patients with alcoholic cirrhosis. Immunology 1981;43:177–182.
9. Fukuda Y, Imoto M, Hayakawa T. Serum levels of secretory immunoglobulin A in liver disease. Am J Gastroenterol 1985;80:237–241.
10. Houseley J. Alpha-2 macroglobulin levels in disease in man. J Clin Pathol 1968;21:27–33.
11. Gjone E, Norum KR. Plasma lecithin-cholesterol acyltransferase and erythrocyte lipid in liver disease. Acta Med Scand 1970;187:153–161.
12. Kindmark CO, Laurell CB. Sequential changes of the plasma protein pattern in inoculation hepatitis. Scand J Clin Lab Invest 1972;29;[Suppl]124:105–115.
13. Fenoglio C, Ferenczy A, Isobe T, Osserman EF. Hepatoma associated with marked plasmacytosis and polyclonal hypergammaglobulinemia. Am J Med 1973;55:111–115.
14. Demenlenaere L, Wieme RJ. Special electrophoretic anomalies in the serum of liver patients: a report of 1145 cases. Am J Dig Dis 1961;6:661–675.
15. Robson AM, Loney LC. Nephrotic syndrome. In: Conn RB, ed. Current diagnosis. Philadelphia: WB Saunders, 1985;7:1102–1108.
16. Whicher JT. The interpretation of electrophoresis. Br J Hosp Med 1980; October:348–360.
17. Appel GB, Blum CB, Chien S, Kunis CL, Appel AS. The hyperlipidemia of the

nephrotic syndrome relation to plasma albumin concentration, oncotic pressure and viscosity. N Engl J Med 1985;312:1544–1548.

18. Keren DF. Whipple's disease. In: Conn RB, ed. Current diagnosis. Philadelphia: WB Saunders, 1985;7:669–671.
19. Schofield KP, Voulgari F, Gozzard DI. C-reactive protein concentrations as a guide to antibiotic therapy in acute leukemia. J Clin Pathol 1982;35:866–869.
20. Ramos CE, Tapia RH. C-reactive protein. Lab Med 1984;16:737–739.
21. Fischer CL, Gill C, Forrester MG, Nakamura R. Quantitation of acute phase proteins postoperatively; value in detection of complications. Am J Clin Pathol 1976;66:840–846.
22. Killingsworth LM. Plasma protein patterns in health and disease. CRC Crit Rev Clin Lab Sci 1979;3:1–30.
23. Smith SJ, Bos G, Esseveld MR, Van Eijk HG, Gerbrandy J. Acute phase proteins from the liver and enzymes from myocardial infarction: a quantitative relationship. Clin Chim Acta 1977;81:75–85.
24. Cooper EH, Stone J. Acute phase reactant proteins in cancer. Adv Cancer Res 1979;30:1–44.
25. Ward AM, Cooper EH. Acute phase proteins in the staging and monitoring of malignancy. Ric Clin Lab 1978;8;[Suppl]1:49–52.
26. Thompson DK, Haddow JE, Smith DE, Ritchie RF. Elevated serum acute phase protein levels as predictors of disseminated breast cancer. Cancer 1983;51:2100–2104.
27. Stava Z. Serum proteins in scleroderma. Dermatologica 1958;117:147–153.
28. Lebac E, Tirzonalis A, Gossart J. Electrophoresis of blood proteins in collagen diseases. Acta Gastroenterol Belg 1959;22:544–549.
29. Killingsworth LM, Yount WJ, Roberts JE. Protein profiles in the rheumatic diseases. Clin Chem 1975;21:1921.
30. Ganrot PO. Variation of the concentrations of some plasma proteins in normal adults, in pregnant women and in newborns. Scand J Clin Lab Invest 1972;29;[Suppl]124:83–88.
31. Burnett D, Wood SM, Bradwell AR. Plasma protein profiles of serum and amniotic fluid in normal pregnancy and preeclampsia. In Peeters H, ed. Protides of the biological fluids (23rd Colloquim, 1975). Oxford: Pergamon, 1976;349–362.
32. Kabat EA, Landow H, Moore DH. Electrophoretic patterns of concentrated cerebrospinal fluid. Proc Soc Exp Biol Med 1942;49:260–263.
33. Kabat EA, Moore DH, Landow H. An electrophoretic study of the protein components in cerebrospinal fluid and their relationship to the serum proteins. J Clin Invest 1942;21:571–577.
34. Jepperson JO, Laurell CB, Franzen B. Agarose gel electrophoresis. Clin Chem 1979;25:629–638.
35. Killingsworth LM, Cooney SK, Tyllia MM, Killingsworth CE. Protein analysis. Deciphering cerebrospinal fluid patterns. Diagn Med 1980;3/4:23–29.
36. Lubahn DB, Silverman LM. A rapid silver-stain procedure for use with routine electrophoresis of cerebrospinal fluid on agarose gels. Clin Chem 1984;30:1689–1691.
37. Mehta PD, Mehta SP, Patrick BA. Silver staining of unconcentrated cerebrospinal fluid in agarose gel (Panagel) electrophoresis. Clin Chem 1984;30:735–736.
38. Parker WC, Bearn AG. Studies of the transferrins of adult serum, cord serum, and cerebrospinal fluid. The effect of neuraminidase. J Exp Med 1962;115:83–93.

39. Wieme RJ. Agar gel electrophoresis. Amsterdam: Elsevier, 1965.

40. Parker WC, Hagstrom J, Bearn AG. Additional studies on the transferrins of cord serum and cerebrospinal fluid. J Exp Med 1963;118:975-983.

41. Laurell DB. Composition and variation of the gel electrophoretic fractions of plasma, cerebrospinal fluid and urine. Scand J Clin Lab Invest 1972;29; [Suppl]124:71-82.

42. Link H. Immunoglobulin G and low molecular weight proteins in human CSF. Acta Neurol Scand 1967;43;[Suppl]28:1-134.

43. Poser CM. Multiple sclerosis and other diseases of the white matter. In Conn RB, ed. Current diagnosis. Philadelphia: WB Saunders, 1985;7:996-1006.

44. Farrell MA, Kaufmann JCE, Gilbert JJ, Noseworthy JH, Armstrong HA, Ebers GC. Oligoclonal bands in multiple sclerosis: clinical-pathologic correlation. Neurology (NY) 1985;35:212-218.

45. Link H, Tibbling G. Principles of albumin and IgG analyses in neurological disorders. III. Evaluation of IgG synthesis within the central nervous system in multiple sclerosis. Scand J Clin Lab Invest 1977;37:397-401.

46. Hershey LA, Trotter JL. The use and abuse of the cerebrospinal fluid IgG profile in the adult: a practical evaluation. Ann Neurol 1980;8:426-434.

47. Lowenthal A, Vansande M, Karcher D. The differential diagnosis of neurological disease by fractionating electrophoretically the CSF-globulins. J Neurochem 1960;6:51-58.

48. Vandvik B, Natvig JB, Wiger D. IgG1 subclass restriction of oligoclonal IgG from cerebrospinal fluids and brain extracts in patients with multiple sclerosis and subacute encephalitis. Scand J Immunol 1976;5:427-436.

49. Jozefczyk PB, Kelly RH, Rabin BS. Clinical significance of immunologic and immunogenetic evaluation in multiple sclerosis. Immunol Commun 1984;13: 371-379.

50. Keshgegian AA, Coblentz J, Lisak RP. Oligoclonal immunoglobulins in cerebrospinal fluid in multiple sclerosis. Clin Chem 1980;26:1340-1345.

51. Ford HC. Abnormalities of serum and plasma components in patients with multiple sclerosis. Clin Biochem 1985;18:3-13.

52. Embers GC, Paty DW. CSF electrophoresis in one thousand patients. Can J Neurol Sci 1980;7:275-280.

53. Keshgegian AA. Cerebrospinal fluid immunoglobulins in multiple sclerosis. Am Assn Clin Chem Specific Protein Analysis 1983;1:1-7.

54. Gerson B, Krolikowski FJ, Gerson IM. Two agarose electrophoretic systems for demonstration of oligoclonal bands in cerebrospinal fluid compared. Clin Chem 1980;26:343-345.

55. Sandberg-Wollheim M. Optic neuritis: studies on the cerebrospinal fluid in relation to clinical course in 61 patients. Acta Neurol Scand 1975;52:167-178.

56. Nikoskelainen E, Frey H, Salmi A. Prognosis of optic neuritis with special reference to cerebrospinal fluid immunoglobulins and measles virus antibodies. Ann Neurol 1981;9:545-550.

57. Gerson B, Cohen SR, Gerson IM, Guest GH. Myelin basic protein, oligoclonal bands and IgG in cerebrospinal fluid as indicators of multiple sclerosis. Clin Chem 1981;27:1974-1977.

58. Bloomer LC, Bray PF. Relative value of three laboratory methods in the diagnosis of multiple sclerosis. Clin Chem 1981;27:2011-2013.

59. Olsson JE, Link H. Immunoglobulin abnormalities in multiple sclerosis. Arch Neurol 1973;28:392–399.

60. Nilsson K, Olsson JE. Analysis for cerebrospinal proteins by isoelectric focusing of polyacrylamide gel: methodological aspects and normal values with special reference to the alkaline region. Clin Chem 1978;24:1134–1139.

61. Cohen SR, Herndon RM, McKahnn GM. Radioimmunoassay of myelin basic protein in spinal fluid: an index of active demyelination. N Engl J Med 1976;295:1455–1457.

62. Whitaker JN, Lisch RP, Bashir RM. Immunoreactive myelin basic protein in the cerebrospinal fluid in neurological disorders. Ann Neurol 1980;7:58–64.

63. Papadopoulos NM, Costello R, Kay AD, Cutler NR, Rapoport SI. Combined immunochemical and electrophoretic determinations of proteins in paired serum and cerebrospinal fluid samples. Clin Chem 1984;30:1814–1816.

64. Dubois EL, Tuffanelli DL. Clinical manifestations of systemic lupus erythematosus: computer analysis of 520 cases. JAMA 1964;190:104–111.

65. Johnson RT, Richardson EP. The neurological manifestations of systemic lupus erythematosus. Medicine 1968;47:337–369.

66. Dubois EL, Wierzchowiecki M, Cox MB. Duration and death in systemic lupus erythematosus: an analysis of 249 cases. JAMA 1974;227:1399–1402.

67. Small P, Mass MF, Kohler PF, Jarbeck RJ. Central nervous system involvement in SLE diagnostic profile and clinical features. Arthritis Rheum 1977;20:869–878.

68. Winfield JB, Shaw M, Silverman LM, Eisenberg RA, Wilson III HA, Koffler D. Intrathecal IgG synthesis and blood–brain barrier impairment in patients with systemic lupus erythematosus and central nervous system dysfunction. Am J Med 1983;74:837–844.

69. Cooper EH, Morgan CB. Proteinuria. Am Assn Clin Chem Specific Protein Analysis 1984;1:1–11.

70. Wieme RJ. Agar gel electrophoresis. Amsterdam: Elsevier, 1965.

71. Yu H, Yanagisawa Y, Forbes M, Cooper EH, Crockson RA, MacLennan ICM. Alpha-1 microglobulin: an indicator protein for renal tubular function. J Clin Pathol 1983;36:253–259.

72. Petersen PA. Characteristics of vitamin A-transporting protein complex occurring in human serum. J Biol Chem 1971;246:34–38.

73. Bernard AM, Lauwreys RR. Retinol binding protein in urine: a more practical index than urinary b-2 microglobulin for the routine screening of renal tubular dysfunction. Clin Chem 1981;27:1781–1782.

74. Laurell CB. Electrophoresis, specific protein assays or both in measurement of plasma proteins. Clin Chem 1973;19:99–102.

75. Fleming JJ, Child JA, Cooper EH, Hay AM, Morgan DB, Parapia L. Renal tubular damage without glomerular damage after cytotoxic drugs and aminoglycosides. Biomedicine 1980;33:251–254.

76. Schentag JJ, Plaut ME. Patterns of urinary beta-2 microglobulin excretion by patients treated with aminoglycosides. Kidney Int 1980;17:654–661.

77. Abdurrahman MB, Edington GM. Correlation between proteinuria selectivity index and kidney histology of nephrotic children in Northern Nigeria. J Trop Pediatr 1982;28:124–126.

78. Poortmans J, van Kerchove E. La proteinurie d'effort. Clin Chim Acta 1962;7:229–242.

79. Hemmingsen L, Skaarup P. Urinary excretion of ten plasma proteins in patients with febrile diseases. Acta Med Scan 1977;200:359–364.
80. Jensen H, Henriksen K. Proteinuria in non-renal infectious diseases. Acta Med Scand 1974;196:75–82.
81. Solling J, Solling K, Mogensen CE. Patterns of proteinuria and circulating immune complexes in febrile patients. Acta Med Scand 1982;212:167–169.
82. Killingsworth LM, Conney SK, Tyllia MM. Protein analysis finding clues to disease in urine. Diagn Med 1980; May–June:69–75.
83. Mengoli C, Lechi A, Arosia E, Rizzotti P, Lechi C, Corgnati A, Micciolo R, Pancera P. Contribution of four markers of tubular proteinuria in detecting upper urinary tract infections. A multivariate analysis. Nephron 1982;32:234–238.
84. Deegan MJ. Bence Jones proteins: nature, metabolism, detection and significance. Ann Clin Lab Sci 1976;6:38–46.

CHAPTER 4

Immunofixation Technique

High-resolution electrophoresis (HRE) allows detection of many more bands in serum, urine, or cerebrospinal fluid than do the older five-band electrophoretic methodologies. This can be a mixed blessing. As is evident from the preceding chapters, identification of individual bands is not always a simple matter. Since the most important reason for performing serum or urine protein electrophoresis is to detect monoclonal proteins indicating the presence of a lymphoplasmacytic neoplastic process, it becomes especially critical to be able to identify suspicious bands. In the clinical laboratories, this identification is most often carried out by performing immunoelectrophoresis (IEP) on the sample. This procedure combines two techniques, electrophoresis and immunoprecipitation, allowing a highly specific identification of suspicious bands. A more rapid and sensitive identification of unknown bands can be achieved by immunofixation, which combines HRE with immunoprecipitation.

PRINCIPLES OF IMMUNOPRECIPITATION

Whether one is performing IEP or immunofixation, the basic principles of the precipitin reaction are the same, and understanding them is critically important to making the correct interpretation of a given sample. Immunoprecipitation involves the interaction of antibody molecules with antigen in either a gel or liquid matrix in which the molecules are free to diffuse. The key to precipitation is the fact that antibodies and antigens each have two or more sites with which they can interact; that is, they are multivalent.

In most chemical reactions, when substance A is mixed with substance B to form a product C (let's call it a precipitate), the reaction can be expressed as

$$A + B \rightarrow C$$

As shown in Figure 4-1, as one increases the amount of substance A with a constant amount of substance B, the amount of precipitate C will increase up to a point and then remains constant despite addition of more substance A because all the available substance B has combined with A to form the pre-

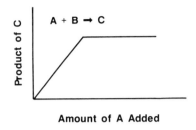

Figure 4–1.   As substance B is used up, no more product C is formed by the addition of substance A.

cipitate. Similarly, in immunologic reactions a precipitable product is formed when an antibody is added to its antigen. Unlike the chemical reaction shown in Figure 4–1, however, a decrease in the amount of precipitate is observed as excess antibody is added to a constant amount of antigen (Figure 4–2). Therefore, there is something about the interaction of antibodies with antigens that differs from the simple chemical reaction shown above.

Antibody–antigen interactions are highly complex because of the many variables that may occur. In the first place, a given antigen molecule has many different surface determinants (epitopes) to which antibodies may bind (Figure 4–3). Each epitope may elicit several different clones of B lymphocytes to differentiate into antibody-secreting plasma cells. The antibodies that are produced by each clone will differ from one another in structure such that their ability to bind to the epitope will vary from one clone to another. This strength of antibody binding to a particular epitope is called the "affinity" and can be expressed mathematically.

The binding of the antibody molecules to epitopes depends on multiple types of noncovalent interactions. The forces involved include:

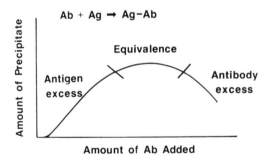

Figure 4–2.   This classic immunoprecipitin curve (Heidelberger curve) shows that the amount of precipitate (antigen–antibody complex) decreases with the addition of excessive amounts of antibody.

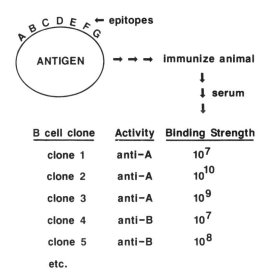

Figure 4-3. Most antigens are complex molecules with many surface epitopes to which antibodies will form. In turn, several different B-cell clones may respond to each epitope, creating a diverse array of antibody specificities of a variety of binding strengths in the reagent antisera that we use.

1. *Coulombic forces,* which result from the interaction of oppositely charged groups such as NH_3^+ with COO^-
2. *Hydrogen bonding,* which results from the interaction of a hydrogen atom that is closely linked to an electronegative atom, such as oxygen, with another electronegative atom
3. *Hydrophobic bonding,* which is analogous to the effects of oil in water. Even when dispersed, the oil will exclude the intervening water molecules and coalesce. Hydrophobic bonding occurs due to the preference of apolar groups for self-association.
4. *Van der Waals forces,* which are interactions that occur in the outer electrons of the reactants. These are relatively weak forces that gain considerably in strength as the antigen and antibody approximate one another.

None of these interactions has the strength of covalent bonding, and therefore antibody–antigen interactions are readily reversible reactions. The strength of the interaction of a particular antibody with a particular epitope (affinity) depends on the number and strength of the four types of bonds described above.

In the immune precipitin reaction, the multivalency of the antibody and antigen allows for the formation of a lattice (Figure 4-4). In the zone of antigen excess (Figure 4-2), the excessive number of antigens present makes it likely that only relatively small immune complexes are formed with the for-

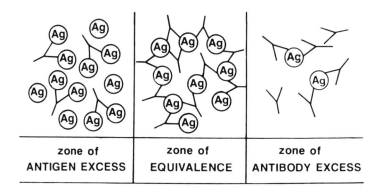

| zone of | zone of | zone of |
| ANTIGEN EXCESS | EQUIVALENCE | ANTIBODY EXCESS |

Figure 4-4. Multivalency of antibody and antigens is responsible for the classic immunoprecipitin curve (Figure 4-2).

mula AB(1)AG(2). These molecules would be too small to form a precipitate. As more antibody is added to the system, a precipitate (large antibody–antigen latticework) begins to form until a maximal precipitate is noted. This maximal precipitate occurs in the zone of equivalence where the formula is AB(1)AG(1) (Figure 4-4). With the addition of more antibody, the epitopes on the surface of the antigen are saturated with antibody molecules and therefore are not available for reaction with other cross-linking antibodies. Here the formula would be AB(x)AG(1) where x = the number of epitopes expressed on the surface of a particular antigen.

Ouchterlony devised a simple way to use the immunoprecipitation reaction to determine antibody reactivity and to identify unknown antigens. He cut wells in an agarose gel and put antibody in one well and antigen in another. These molecules diffuse radially out of the wells (Figure 4-5). As they diffuse

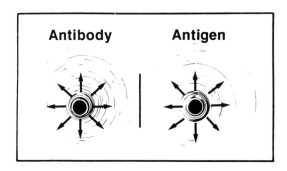

Figure 4-5. As antibody and antigen diffuse from the well, their concentrations decrease logarithmically. The precipitin line forms where the concentrations are equivalent.

away from the center of the well, their concentration decreases logarithmically. A precipitin band forms somewhere between the two wells at the point at which their concentrations are equivalent. If the precipitate is closer to the antigen well, it indicates that the antibody was more concentrated than the antigen because it had to diffuse further than the antigen (thereby becoming more dilute) before a precipitate could be seen. Other factors such as the size of the molecules and their possible interactions with the gel also affect this reaction, but in general the beauty of the antibody–antigen interactions when they diffuse through agarose gel for a distance is that the concentration of the reactants is automatically adjusted to form the precipitate.

Ouchterlony also found that by using a known antigen and antibody he could determine whether an unknown antigen was the same, similar, or dissimilar. In Figure 4–6 are shown the results of using an antiserum that has

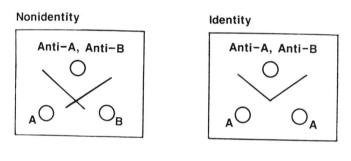

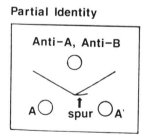

Figure 4–6. Ouchterlony plates using specific antibodies can be used to determine the antigen content of unknown solutions. When different antigens (A and B) are reacted with antibodies to A and B, two lines form, which cross one another (nonidentity). When the antigen in both wells is the same, the two lines meet (identity) because the antibodies to the antigen are absorbed out in the precipitation and do not pass beyond the precipitin line to react with the other antigen. When the antigen is similar (A'), only some of the antibodies to the antigen (A) will be removed. Antibodies to antigen A that are not expressed on A' will pass through the precipitin band formed by anti-A and A', and a second line (spur) will form with antigen A. This is the partial identity pattern.

reactivity with both antigen A and B. If antigen A is in one test well and antigen B is in the other, a pattern of nonidentity occurs where the two lines cross. Some individuals do not understand how the two lines can cross. How do the antibodies to antigen B pass through the precipitin line resulting from the interaction of anti-A with antigen A? Realize that the precipitin line does not resemble a steel wall, but a grossly visible latticework (Figure 4–4). Other antibodies and antigens can readily pass through this latticework.

If antigen A is placed in both test wells, a pattern of identity occurs. Here the lines meet but do not cross one another, because all the antibodies to antigen A react with substance A and cannot pass through the lattice. If antigen A is placed in one test well and a chemically similar antigen A' (which may lack one epitope that antigen A possesses) is placed in the other test well, a pattern of partial identity results. This is one of the more difficult patterns to identify and to understand. Here, all of the molecules that react with antigen A' are precipitated onto the lattice when they meet antibody to A. However, since antigen A' lacks one epitope that is present on antigen A, antibodies to this epitope pass through the lattice formed by anti-A + antigen A' and are available to interact with antigen A. Since there are only relatively few of these molecules and most of the antibodies that react with anti-A have been removed by the interaction with A', antigen A must diffuse slightly farther (to become more dilute in concentration) before it is in equivalence to form a precipitate with the fewer remaining anti-A molecules. This explains the "spur" of antigen A, which is the classic definition of "partial identity."

IMMUNOELECTROPHORESIS

Immunoelectrophoresis (IEP) is performed by placing the patient's serum into a well in an agarose gel. The sample is electrophoresed to permit separation of the major serum proteins (Figure 4–7). After electrophoresis, the gel is removed from the electrophoretic apparatus and the troughs are filled with antisera to various specific components of interest, usually including antipolyvalent human immunoglobulin (which reacts with all heavy and light chain classes), anti-IgG, anti-IgA, anti-IgM, antikappa, and antilambda. For comparison, and to insure that the correct antisera has been placed into the appropriate troughs, a control serum is alternated with the patient's sample on the IEP strip. These antisera slowly diffuse into the gel while the protein components slowly diffuse toward the antisera. Precipitin lines form where the antisera and the specific antigens are at equivalence. Due to the geometry of the application wells and radial diffusion, the precipitin lines are in the form of arcs. Large monoclonal proteins are readily identified by IEP by comparing the migration of the control to the patient's serum across a trough containing a specific antiserum (Figure 4–8).

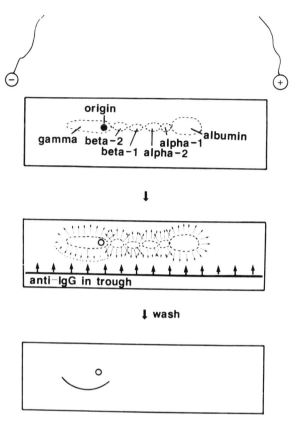

Figure 4-7. Immunoelectrophoresis (IEP) takes advantage of the principles of electrophoresis, gel diffusion (which adjusts concentrations during diffusion), and antibody-antigen precipitin reactions to identify specific proteins. In the example shown, only IgG is precipitated and present after the wash step. The closer the IgG is to the antiserum trough, the greater is its concentration. Large molecules such as pentameric IgM can be difficult to examine by this technique because they diffuse slowly through the agarose. Small monoclonal proteins are also difficult to identify because this technique does not offer good resolution of individual proteins.

The ability to perform IEP was a significant advance in the identification of monoclonal proteins associated with multiple myeloma and Waldenstrom's macroglobulinemia. Unlike nephelometry or immunofixation (see subsequent discussion), it was not necessary to be overly concerned with the antigen excess situation, (that is, one in which the patient has a very large amount of monoclonal protein), because as the protein diffused into the agar, its concentration decreased greatly, allowing the system to automatically adjust to antigen–antibody equivalence and a precipitin arc to be formed. When monoclonal pro-

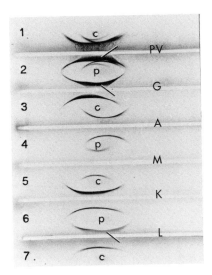

Figure 4-8.   IEP shows a large IgG lambda monoclonal gammopathy. Note that control (c) serum alternates with patient (p) serum. Antisera to polyvalent (PV), IgG (G), IgA (A), IgM (M), kappa (K), and lambda (L) were placed in the troughs. A large arc with excessively anodal migration is seen in the polyvalent, IgG, and lambda areas of the patient's sample (indicated in all three locations). The lambda arc stains weakly, which is the prozone phenomenon often seen with lambda reagents. Diagnosis of such large monoclonal gammopathies is relatively easy by IEP.

teins were found in such great quantities, IEP was still able to diagnose the condition properly because of this diffusion effect. In the latter case the precipitin arc would merely be close to the trough or the center of the arc would actually diffuse into the trough (Figure 4–9).

Similarly, IEP could detect a second monoclonal protein such as a free monoclonal light chain (Bence Jones protein), which may occur simultaneously with an intact monoclonal protein. This was possible because the light chain has a much smaller molecular weight than the intact immunoglobulin molecule and a free light chain has certain epitopes (antigenic determinants) exposed on its surface that are hidden (not on the surface) of an intact immunoglobulin molecule. When commercial antisera are able to detect these epitopes, they have separate reactivity for light chains (Figure 4–10). Consequently, as with the Ouchterlony patterns of partial identity discussed above, when the intact immunoglobulin molecule reacts with the antiserum it cannot remove antibodies to these hidden determinants. The latter antibodies proceed on through to react with the free light chain.

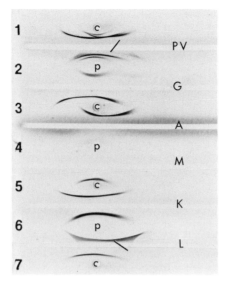

Figure 4-9. IEP of urine shows a large lambda Bence Jones protein. Note that control (c) is serum so that we can see the position of normal IgG, IgA, and IgM. Normal urine would have too little immunoglobulin to detect with this method. The patient's urine (p) has so much of the monoclonal lambda protein that it has substantially diffused into the trough before reaching "equivalence" and forming a precipitate with the antipolyvalent (PV) and antilambda (L) reagents (*indicated*). Note that the polyvalent reaction is quite weak. It is typical for polyvalent reagents to have relatively weak antilambda reactivity. Compare this to Figure 4-8 (symbols are same), in which the dense reaction in the polyvalent reagent is due to the anti-IgG (G) in the polyvalent reagent.

LIMITATIONS OF IMMUNOELECTROPHORESIS

Unfortunately, there are several problems with IEP that encouraged the development of newer approaches to the diagnosis of monoclonal gammopathies. Although IEP is an accurate means to diagnose a large monoclonal gammopathy, it is also very slow, largely because of the diffusion step, which requires at least 18 hours for optimal results. After this, for greatest sensitivity the gel must be washed and stained before final examination. In our laboratory, the typical IEP with no complicating factors takes 3 days to complete.

Besides being slow, IEP is unable to distinguish monoclonality in certain types of monoclonal proteins [1–6]. The case shown in Figure 4–11 is a typical example of the "umbrella effect" problem on IEP. The patient was a 60-year-

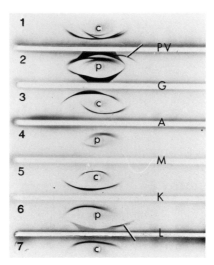

Figure 4-10. IEP from the serum of a patient with both a monoclonal IgG lambda protein and a free lambda monoclonal light chain (Bence Jones protein) in the serum. The free lambda light chain reactivity can be seen with the polyclonal reagent, where the extra arc due to the anti-free lambda is indicated. The same area is indicated in the antilambda reaction with the patient's serum in the bottom trough. This area is not seen with the anti-IgG reagent.

old woman who complained of lethargy and was noted on physical examination to have prominent axillary lymph nodes. Despite an IgM level (1330 mg/dl) greater than three times our upper limit of normal (350 mg/dl) and an obvious spike on serum protein electrophoresis (Figure 4–12), the IEP (Figure 4–11) of this patient's serum was nondiagnostic. One could certainly say that the patient had more IgM than the control, but that was already known from the immunoglobulin quantifications. Monoclonality (marked predominance of kappa or lambda) could not be determined, because the patient had normal amounts of IgG which, with a molecular weight of 160,000, is much smaller than the typical IgM molecule that has a molecular weight of 1,000,000. The smaller molecular weight allows IgG to diffuse more quickly through agarose and to react with antisera to the light chains attached to the IgG, obscuring the light chain type of the bulkier, more slowly diffusing IgM. This masking of an IgM monoclonal gammopathy by polyclonal IgG molecules is called the "umbrella effect," and is a well-known problem in IEP interpretation.

There are several ways that one can still use IEP to make the correct diagnosis in this case [7,8]. One can add 2-mercaptoethanol to break disulfide bonds and then repeat the IEP. Unfortunately, as in this case, this method is sometimes unsuccessful. Reduction of disulfide bonds works best to identify

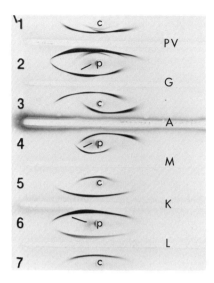

Figure 4-11. Nondiagnostic IEP in a patient with fourfold increase in IgM and an obvious gamma spike on the serum protein electrophoresis (shown on the top of Figure 4-12). The patient's IgM is pentameric and is barely able to migrate out of the well. The diffuse hazy area indicated near the well for all the patient's samples is where the monoclonal protein has deposited. The normal kappa and lambda arcs represent the patient's normal serum IgG and do not reflect his monoclonal protein (so-called "umbrella effect").

those monoclonal IgM proteins that are elevated more than fourfold over normal [8]. Other successful methods involve either a sizing column or a charge column to separate the IgM from the IgG and then repeating the IEP on this separated fraction; methods that are labor intensive and take considerable time, delaying the diagnosis. Such inefficient procedures are also expensive, an even greater problem with modern reimbursement systems, which penalize hospitals for a slow diagnosis. While some have argued that the combined cost of such special procedures with IEP is less than that of immunofixation [8], such has not been our experience. Our costs are detailed in comparison with our IEP costs at the end of this chapter. With immunofixation, one gets the correct result the first time in 1 day. With IEP and special procedures, several days are needed, as the first IEP may be unreadable.

Another difficulty is that the geometry of the IEP setup prevents an optimal resolution of individual protein molecules. Therefore, it can be very difficult to detect biclonal gammopathies, which are readily detected with systems such as immunofixation that allow a greater discrimination between two different monoclonal proteins that have relatively close pI (see Chapter 1).

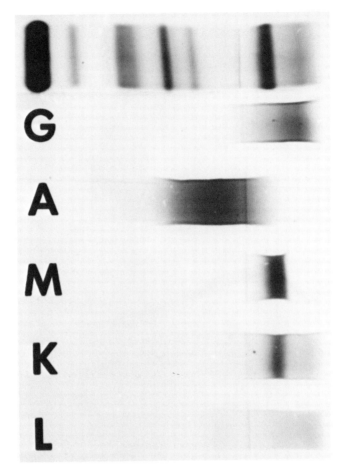

Figure 4–12. Immunofixation of serum from Figure 4–11. Top sample is just HRE of patient's serum run at same time as immunofixation. After electrophoresis, it was cut from the gel, fixed, and stained as described later. Cellulose acetate strips with 50 μl of antisera to IgG (G), IgA (A), IgM (M), kappa (K), and lambda (L) were placed directly onto the agarose gels in the indicated positions. After staining, the interpretation is an obvious IgM kappa monoclonal gammopathy. Note that the monoclonal protein has the same electrophoretic migration in the reaction with anti-IgM and antikappa. Also, by using the serum at the proper dilution (*see text*), you have a built-in control for the antisera. IgA reacts in a broad beta region where IgA normally migrates. Similarly, anti-IgG and antilambda reagents show proper reactivity.

IEP lacks sensitivity to detect smaller monoclonal gammopathies. Some believe that this insensitivity of IEP is an advantage because the larger monoclonal gammopathies detected are more likely to be of clinical significance than smaller monoclonal gammopathies. Experienced practitioners of clinical and laboratory medicine know, however, that ignorance is rarely equated with bliss for long. In recent years, it has become clear that small monoclonal gammopathies are important to detect. It is true that often we do not yet understand the clinical significance for the particular patient. Indeed, Kyle [9] has coined the appropriate term "monoclonal gammopathy of undetermined significance" for such patients. However, those patients need to be followed as the gammopathy may develop into a malignant monoclonal process (myeloma, Waldenstrom's), or small monoclonal gammopathies may represent the presence of a malignant B-cell neoplasm (see Chapter 5). Such small monoclonal gammopathies have now been found in chronic lymphocytic leukemia, Burkitt's lymphoma, and in well-differentiated lymphocytic lymphoma [10–12]. Also, it has become clear that many patients with neurologic complaints have monoclonal gammopathies that are related to their clinical symptoms [13–15].

Detection of these small monoclonal gammopathies requires that more sensitive techniques than routine IEP be used. In the past, when small monoclonal gammopathies were suspected due to the presence of a restricted band on serum protein electrophoresis, our laboratory would spend several days, often a week or more, trying to purify this protein by column techniques, then concentrating the purified protein and performing IEP to identify it.

IMMUNOFIXATION

Immunofixation has been a dramatic new development for the clinical laboratory in the past few years [16–20). This technique can be performed from start to finish in 1 day, is not subject to the umbrella effect, can readily detect the small monoclonal gammopathies that may accompany B-cell neoplasms, is easier to interpret than IEP, uses half as much antisera as IEP, and requires the same equipment as that needed for HRE.

The decision as to whether or not immunofixation is required rests with those who understand the capabilities and the problems of the techniques— the clinical laboratory. Our strategies for dealing with various clinical requests are detailed in Chapter 5. When we have determined that immunofixation should be performed, we use the same electrophoretic apparatus that was described for HRE in Chapter 1. Electrophoretic systems available from many commercial suppliers permit the laboratory to perform immunofixation on either agarose or cellulose acetate.

The patient's sample is set up as shown in Figure 4–12. It is critically important to know the concentrations of the major immunoglobulin classes before one sets up the immunofixation plate. With most commercial antisera, the antigen (IgG, IgA, IgM, kappa, or lambda) to be precipitated needs to be about 100 mg/dl for an optimal precipitation. With IEP it was not necessary to adjust the concentration of the patient's serum because the slow diffusion step allowed this to occur automatically. However, in immunofixation the diffusion area is minimal and the diffusion step is rapid. Therefore, there is not sufficient diffusion to allow the concentration of the antigen and antibody to adjust to equivalence for maximal precipitation.

Fortunately, adjustment for concentration is relatively simple. For example, with the immunoglobulin values shown in Table 4-1 and in most clinical laboratories, results are expressed as mg/100 ml. To determine the appropriate dilution to use for a given sample, divide the quantity of the immunoglobulin by 100. If the number is less than 1, the serum should be undiluted (neat). Note that the optimal dilution will vary somewhat between different antisera. The 100 mg/dl is a useful approximation for most which we have used.

$$\text{Dilution of serum for IgX} = \frac{\text{Igx}}{100}$$

A separate sample of patient serum appropriately diluted must be applied to the gel for each immunoglobulin or other antigen to be assayed. Usually, one prepares the immunofixation for IgG, IgA, IgM, kappa, and lambda (Figure 4-12). However, IgE, IgD, or other antigens such as C-reactive protein may be useful for specific samples (Chapter 6). Additionally, a sample of the patient's serum should be run in parallel; this will be used as the HRE standard.

Following electrophoresis, the HRE standard strip is fixed with acid (Chapter 1). In some systems such as the one we use, this is accomplished by cutting out the strip and processing it as in Chapter 1. Other systems allow one to simply overlay the strip with fixative to precipitate the serum proteins. For specific immunoglobulins, the patient's sample is overlain with a strip of celluose acetate onto which 50 μl of specific antiserum have been placed. This strip is placed directly on top of the electrophoresed sample. Since the diffusion is directly into the thin gel beneath, only 1 hour is required. Following this step, the gels are washed and stained with Coomassie blue (which we prefer) or Amido black (Chapter 1). Some workers have used silver staining for enhanced sensitivity, but because in our hands the commercially available silver stains have been difficult to use and have provided us with so much back-

Table 4-1   Calculation of Dilution of Serum to Use with Immunofixation

Immunoglobulin	Concentration (mg/dl)	Dilution[a]
IgG	1434	1:14
IgA	241	1:2
IgM	126	Undiluted
Kappa-containing	1047	1:10
Lambda-containing	683	1:7

[a]Dilution is based on closest approximation to 100 mg/dl. If antigen excess effect is seen, a greater dilution of serum will be needed for your system. We have found this to be needed with antilambda reagents.

ground that the overall interpretation was more difficult, we recommend the simpler Coomassie blue technique.

Interpretation of immunofixation patterns is accomplished by lining up the stained HRE strip of the patient's serum with the stained immunofixation gel (Figure 4-12). The suspected monoclonal band in the patient's serum will have the same electrophoretic mobility in the immunofixation gel as it does in the HRE strip. Therefore, one looks down the gel and finds the location of the precipitin lines. This indicates the specific monoclonal protein. It is important that the monoclonal protein line up with the suspected band as other proteins such as C-reactive protein can (albeit rarely) account for a suspicious band in a HRE. When two or more small bands are detected, one is usually dealing with an oligoclonal expansion in a patient with an infectious disease or an autoimmune disease with polyclonal expansion of immunoglobulins (Figure 4-13). Biclonal gammopathies do occur and can be readily diagnosed by immunofixation (Figure 4-14). They are usually simple to distinguish from the polyclonal process shown in Figure 4-13. The monoclonal proteins are in greater concentration than those of the polyclonal processes, and often there is an accompanying decrease in concentration of the other immunoglobulins as opposed to the diffuse increase of other immunoglobulins that accompanies polyclonal processes (Figure 4-14). Because of the high resolution achieved with the electrophoresis, two monoclonal proteins with relatively close isoelectric points can be detected, whereas such discrimination often was not possible with IEP.

Unlike IEP, where a small monoclonal protein is difficult to discern and often requires considerable experience and laborious time-consuming procedures to detect, immunofixation allows rapid correct diagnosis of small monoclonal gammopathies by even inexperienced workers. For example, the small monoclonal gammopathy in Figure 4-15 is obvious by immunofixation but was not detected by IEP. Its detection by IEP required column purification, concentration, and repeated IEP, which delay diagnosis for as much as a week.

A common problem with IEP of proteins with large molecular weights, such as IgM or occasionally IgA (which also occurs as polymers), is the umbrella effect. Due to the rapid diffusion step and better resolution of individual proteins, no umbrella effect is seen with immunofixation. This alone has saved us several days in diagnosis of specific samples and saved considerably in reagent cost and technologist time.

LIMITATIONS OF IMMUNOFIXATION

There are elements of immunofixation technique of which the reader must be aware to avoid common errors. First, because of the rapid diffusion step, the monoclonal protein cannot automatically adjust its concentration as was true in IEP. Therefore, dilution of the patient's sample for each immunoglobulin assayed is a critically important step. For instance, when a large amount of

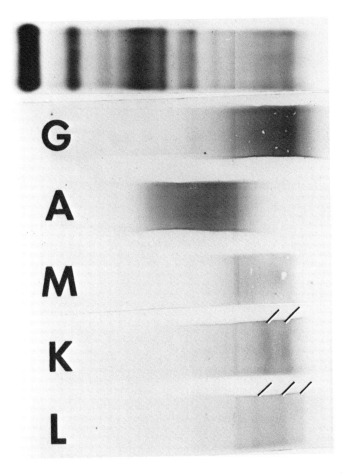

Figure 4-13. Immunofixation of serum of patient with pneumonia who had a few (oligoclonal) bands in the gamma region of HRE. Immunofixation shows that the bands are both kappa and lambda, therefore polyclonal. Some of the small, round, clear areas seen best in the anti-IgG and anti-IgM reaction are caused by air bubbles that prevent the precipitin reaction from occurring. (Symbols as in Figure 4-12.)

monoclonal protein is present, an antigen excess effect can be seen (Figure 4-16). In antigen excess, the immune complexes formed are small and will wash away in steps subsequent to the immunofixation. Similarly, if relatively little immunoglobulin of one class is present, this must be taken into account or one will be in antibody excess with a similar result.

Unfortunately, in an attempt to simplify the method, some commercial manufacturers recommend a standard dilution for IgG, IgA, and IgM. While this standard dilution will work most of the time, it will clearly cause misinterpretation of some samples. The problem with such oversimplification is that

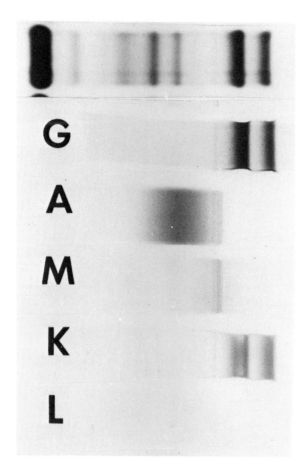

Figure 4–14. Electrophoresis of this sample shows two distinct gamma bands identified as IgGL by immunofixation. The two bands may reflect a monoclonal protein that forms monomers and dimers or may be a true double (biclonal) gammopathy. In this case, subclass determination showed that the two bands were of different subclasses of IgG (a double gammopathy). Unlike Figure 4–13, which shows a diffuse increase in the IgG proteins due to an infectious process, there is a relatively clear background in the gamma area of this immunofixation. The origin artifact in the IgA and IgM reactions is seen in some monoclonal proteins, which tend to self-aggregate. It is most obvious in the IgA and IgM reactions here because the serum samples were applied undiluted to the gel (since the IgA and IgM concentrations were low). However, this optimizes conditions for self-aggregation, and the monoclonal protein gave a visible precipitate at the origin. If this sample were run without anti-A or anti-M, the origin artifact would still be present as it reflects self-aggregation of the monoclonal protein and is not a true immune precipitate. (Symbols as in Figure 4–12.)

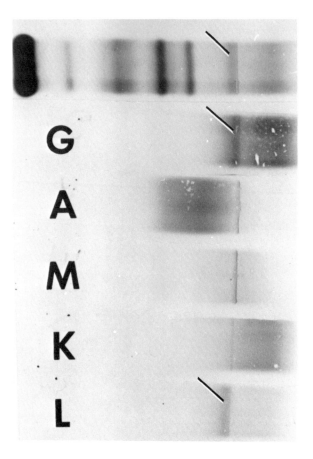

Figure 4-15. This pattern shows a small restriction (*indicated*) just slightly anodal to the origin. The same restriction can be seen in the IgG and lambda precipitin reactions (*indicated*). Note that two artifacts are present in this sample. The holes, representing air-bubble artifacts and the slight origin restriction in the IgA and IgM reactions, occur because the serum is applied undiluted at these sites. Even though the reaction is near the origin, the difference in migration of this origin artifact from the true precipitin bands in IgG and lambda is obvious. (Symbols as in Figure 4-12.)

it ignores the importance of the classic Heidelberger precipitin curve (Figure 4-2). Although immunofixation changes the geometry and simplifies the interpretation, it does not change the basics of antibody–antigen interactions discussed previously in this chapter. To avoid this dilemma, we suggest following the strategies outlined in Chapter 5 for handling samples suspected of having monoclonal proteins; first perform HRE to determine if a suspicious band is present and also perform quantification of IgG, IgA, IgM, kappa, and lambda. Since this must be done before immunofixation, one already knows the quan-

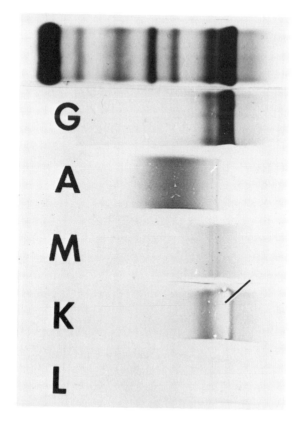

Figure 4–16. HRE shows a large gamma spike. It is obvious from the immunofixation that this is an IgG spike. However, the light chain is not as readily seen, because the wrong dilution of serum was placed in the kappa reaction. Too much kappa-containing immunoglobulin was present, which created an antigen-excess situation. The small complexes formed were removed during the wash step, leaving the clear area indicated. Note that it is surrounded by kappa, which was present at a lower concentration. (Symbols as in Figure 4–12.)

tities of antigen (each immunoglobulin class) and the adjustment can easily be made.

The reader will notice that whereas IEP has a control serum sample alternating with the patient's sample, allowing for comparison across the specific antibody trough, immunofixation does not routinely employ a control serum. If the appropriate dilution of the serum is used, the normal immunoglobulins for each class should be precipitated along with the monoclonal protein. As shown in Figure 4–17, a normal serum should have a precipitate for each immunoglobulin class. This is not background. This precipitate represents the normal immunoglobulin of the isotype for which you are testing.

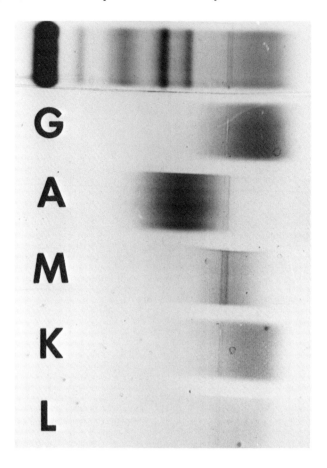

Figure 4-17. Normal HRE and immunofixation. Note origin artifact with undiluted IgM. (Symbols as in Figure 4-12.)

For instance, note that the IgA in Figure 4-17 gives a diffuse staining in the beta region, because IgA is mainly a beta-migrating globulin. Similarly, IgM stays near the origin and IgG is mainly a gamma-migrating globulin.

If one uses a "standard" dilution for all samples, often no precipitin line will be seen (Figure 4-18). When no precipitin line or haze is seen, how do you know that the correct antiserum was actually placed onto the gel or added to the cellulose acetate strip? To optimize the detection of monoclonal proteins and for a built-in control of the methodology, the correct dilution of the patient's serum must be used.

Immunofixation is, however, well worth performing because the high resolution affords sufficient separation of the monoclonal protein allowing its detection even when present in relatively small quantities (Figure 4-15). Such

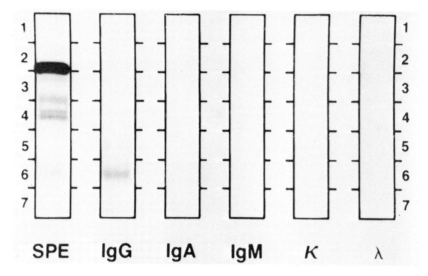

Figure 4-18. Standard dilution recommended by manufacturer shows a restricted band in IgG but no light chain to correspond. Also, was antisera actually placed onto the trough? There is no control, so you do not know unless you see the normal precipitin areas.

subtle shifts could only be detected by IEP when a control serum was run for comparison, and even then further purification steps were usually necessary. Further, with immunofixation, the patient's own sample provides a built-in reagent control.

Some workers claim that too many "unimportant" bands are detected with immunofixation that would not be visible with IEP. It is true that immunofixation is so sensitive that one can often see oligoclonal bands as described above in patients with infectious or autoimmune disease. Occasionally, one of these bands will be rather prominent and one may be tempted to call it a small monoclonal protein. Experience with interpreting these patterns together with some reasonable common sense will prevent any serious overinterpretation. With a difficult case, it may be best to suggest that the clinician repeat the immunofixation in 6 months to determine if the process resolves (which would be the case in the typical infection), stays the same (as may occur in a monoclonal gammopathy of undetermined significance or an autoimmune process that remains active), or progresses (as may occur in early myeloma or Waldenstrom's macroglobulinemia). However, most cases can be resolved by speaking to the clinician about the clinical situation.

Immunofixation is not able to detect some subtle reactivities in human serum that can occur under special circumstances. One such circumstance that we have observed is that of anti-bovidae antibodies in patients with IgA deficiency. Individuals with IgA deficiency often develop antibodies to bovidae protein, presumably from oral stimulation by cow's milk. Since bovidae proteins also are found in goat and sheep serum (often sources of commercial antisera), a peculiar reactivity was often seen by radial immunodiffusion or IEP when testing such serum. Although this antibody did not have clinical significance, it would often be misinterpreted as serum IgA, thus obscuring the patient's IgA deficiency.

Because of the enhanced sensitivity and resolution of immunofixation, minor antibody reactivities in reagent antisera can create potentially confusing patterns. Most commercial antisera are monospecific reagents for the stated immunoglobulin. We test all such sera on receipt, and most have the reactivity stated. However, in our hands, many reagents have minor cross-reactivities with some other serum proteins. The most common such reactivity seen has been with beta-region-migrating proteins, especially C3. This has been found most frequently with anti-IgM and anti-IgA reagents (Figure 4–19). Reactivity with fibrinogen, C4, and transferrin can also occur. Usually, this reaction is seen when the sample is run undiluted. The lack of reactivity with the other reagents should cause the interpreter to suspect this cross-reactivity. Quality control of such reagents should include use of a normal serum run undiluted for immunofixation.

COST CONSIDERATIONS

Overall, immunofixation has proven to be a more rapid, reliable, and sensitive method to detect clinically significant monoclonal proteins in a wide variety of patients. Assuming that only one test is being run (obviously the most inefficient situation), our direct cost analysis of this assay includes the following:

Technologist time—40 min	$ 7.19
Fringe benefits	1.37
Materials (including gel, antisera, pipettes, buffers, blotters, tubes, stain)	13.60
	$ 22.16

The assay is performed and read in 1 day. When monoclonal proteins are identified, the clinician is immediately informed. Our IEP assay had the following direct cost analysis:

Technologist time—40 min	$ 7.19
Fringe benefits	1.37
Materials (including gel, antisera, pipettes, buffers, blotters, tubes, stain)	12.75
	$ 21.31

With immunofixation, we can detect small monoclonal proteins and those affected by the umbrella effect, which resulted in our repeating IEP after var-

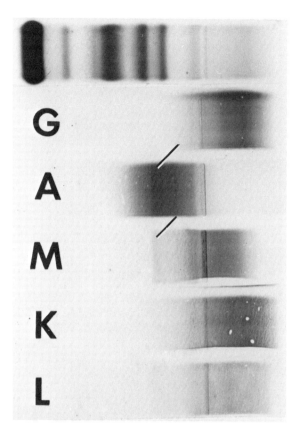

Figure 4-19.   HRE shows normal pattern with a faint fibrinogen band seen just anodal to the origin. The anti-IgA and anti-IgM reactions show a faint but distinct band (*indicated*) due to reactivity of these commercial antisera with C3 in this case. Minor reactivities such as these usually were too dilute to be noticed with IEP. They can be controlled for by testing reagents with a normal serum prior to use with patient samples. Such controls should also be run for IEP. (Symbols as in Figure 4-12.)

ious purification procedures. Lastly, immunofixation can be performed in less than 1 day, while IEP requires at least 2 days. If even a small number of patients have their hospital stay shortened by performing immunofixation, this alone makes the system worthwhile for both the patient and the hospital.

REFERENCES

1.   Smith AM, Thompson RA, Haeney MR. Detection of monoclonal immunoglobulins by immunoelectrophoresis: a possible source of error. J Clin Pathol 1980;33:500–504.

2. Reichert CM, Evertt Jr DF, Nadler, PI, Papadopoulos NM. High-resolution zone electrophoresis, combined with immunofixation, in the detection of an occult myeloma protein. Clin Chem 1982;28:2312–2313.
3. Whicher JT, Chambers RE. Immunofixation can replace immunoelectrophoresis. Clin Chem 1984;30:1112–1113.
4. Aguzzi F, Kohn J, Merlini G, Riches PG. More on immunofixation vs. immunoelectrophoresis. Clin Chem 1984;30:1113.
5. Pudek MR. Investigation of monoclonal gammopathies by immunoelectrophoresis and immunofixation. Clin Chem 1982;28:1231–1232.
6. Ritchie RF, Smith R. Immunofixation. III. Application to the study of monoclonal proteins. Clin Chem 1976;22:1982–1985.
7. Lane JR, Bowles KJ, Normansell DE. Detection of IgM monoclonal proteins in serum enhanced by removal of IgG. Lab Med 1985;16:676–678.
8. Normansell DE. Comparison of five methods for the analysis of the light chain type of monoclonal serum IgM proteins. Am J Clin Pathol 1985;84:469–475.
9. Kyle RA. The monoclonal gammopathies. Springfield: Charles C. Thomas, 1976.
10. Deegan MJ, Abraham JP, Sawdyk M, Van Slyck EJ. High incidence of monoclonal proteins in the serum and urine of chronic lymphocytic leukemia patients. Blood 1984;6:1207–1211.
11. Qian G, Fu SM, Solanki DL, Rai KR. Circulating monoclonal IgM proteins in B-cell chronic lymphocytic leukemia: their identification, characterization and relationship to membrane IgM. J Immunol 1984;133:3396–3400.
12. Braunstein AH, Keren DF. Monoclonal gammopathy (IgM-kappa) occurring in Burkitt's lymphoma. Arch Pathol Lab Med 1983;107:235–238.
13. Steck AJ, Murray N, Meier C, Page N, Perrusseau G. Demyelinating neuropathy and monoclonal IgM antibody to myelin-associated glycoprotein. Neurology 1983;33:19–23.
14. Driedger H, Pruzanski W. Plasma cell neoplasia with peripheral neuropathy. Medicine 1980;59:301–310.
15. Dalakas MC, Engel WK. Polyneuropathy with monoclonal gammopathy: studies of 11 patients. Ann Neurol 1981;10:45–52.
16. Ritchie RF, Smith R. Immunofixation. I. General principles and application to agarose gel electrophoresis. Clin Chem 1976;22:497–499.
17. Sun T, Lien Y, Kunins M. Comparison of immunoelectrophoresis (IEP) and immunofixation (IF) technique in the study of monoclonal gammopathy. Clin Chem 1977;23:1154–1155.
18. Cawley LP, Minard BJ, Toutellotte WW, Ma BI, Chelle C. Immunofixation electrophoretic techniques applied to identification of proteins in serum and cerebrospinal fluid. Clin Chem 1976;22:1262–1268.
19. Vartdal F, Vandvik B. Characterization of classes of intrathecally synthesized antibodies by imprint immunofixation of electrophoretically separated sera and cerebrospinal fluids. Acta Path Microbiol Immunol Scand [Suppl] (C) 1983;91:69–75.
20. Janik B. Identification of monoclonal proteins by immunofixation. Electrophoresis Today 1981;2:1–4.

CHAPTER 5

Strategies for Diagnosing Monoclonal Gammopathies

Monoclonal gammopathies result from many more conditions than just multiple myeloma. In all causes of monoclonal gammopathies, the "M" component derives from a single clone of relatively mature B lymphocytes or plasma cells. The term M component has several definitions in the literature: monoclonal protein, myeloma protein, and macroglobulin [1]. Regardless of the condition behind the monoclonal component (M component) in any particular case, the lesion reflects an aberration of the normal maturation scheme of B lymphocytes to plasma cells. In this chapter we review the development of B lymphocytes and their plasma cell progeny, the clinical pictures associated with monoclonal gammopathies, and strategies for diagnosing monoclonal gammopathies, which include the use of high-resolution electrophoresis (HRE), immunoglobulin quantification, and immunofixation. These methodologies allow the diagnosis of many monoclonal gammopathies in 1 day.

ONTOGENY OF B LYMPHOCYTES

The discovery that there are major subpopulations of lymphocytes resulted from careful observations of immune deficiency in humans and a serendipitous discovery in bursectomized chickens. In 1952, Bruton [2] described a child with recurrent infections of pyogenic bacteria. By using serum protein electrophoresis, then a relatively new clinical laboratory test, he demonstrated that the gamma globulin region was absent in that patient. The patient was treated successfully by administering gamma globulin parenterally. Such patients are now known to have Bruton's X-linked agammaglobulinemia, which is due to a deficient maturation of the B lymphocytes. A few years later, Glick et al. [3] discovered that chickens whose cloacal bursa was removed early in life also developed agammaglobulinemia like the Bruton's patients. Both these chickens and the individuals with Bruton's agammaglobulinemia lacked plasma cells in their tissues, and neither had germinal centers in their lymphoid tissues.

Nonetheless, abundant numbers of lymphocytes were present in these patients, and they had no clinical problems with viral, fungal, or intracellular bacterial infections. We know today that these remaining lymphocytes were T (thymus-derived) lymphocytes, which play the main role in host defense against viral, fungal, and intracellular bacterial infections.

B lymphocytes are so named because in the chicken they are derived from the Bursa of Fabricius. Unfortunately, the literature has been sullied with the term "bone-marrow-derived" lymphocytes in humans as being the equivalent of B cells in the chicken, which is incorrect. Both B and T cells originate in the bone marrow. However, T cells must be processed subsequently in the thymus gland. It is not clear where B lymphocytes are subsequently processed in humans. Therefore, a more correct meaning for "B" cells in humans (for those too proud to recognize their distant relationship to the chicken?) would be "bursal-equivalent" cells, as humans do not have a bursa of Fabricius. Several earlier theories that Peyer's patches and/or the appendix were bursa-like primary lymphoid tissues were also not true. All human gut-associated lymphoid tissues (Peyer's patches, isolated lymphoid follicles, and the appendix) are secondary lymphoid structures roughly equivalent in function to lymph nodes or the spleen, except that they preferentially respond with an IgA rather than IgG plasma cell proliferation when challenged by antigen.

Although the earliest stage of B-lymphocyte development occurs in the fetal liver and bone marrow, this development continues in adult life in the bone marrow (Figure 5-1) [4]. Early on, these cells can be detected by virtue of their expression of the CALLA antigen (common acute lymphocytic leukemia antigen) and the presence of the enzyme terminal deoxyribonucleotidyl transferase in the nucleus (Figure 5-1). At this time, these primitive B cells have already rearranged their mu chain gene, although the mu heavy chain cannot yet be detected in the cytoplasm [5,6]. These "pre-pre-B" cells usually express the Ia antigen and have surface markers for the commercially available monoclonal antibodies B1 and B4 [7].

Around the eighth week of human gestation, large lymphoid cells with a small amount of detectable cytoplasmic mu chain but no detectable light chain are seen in the fetal liver. These have been termed "pre-B" cells [8,9], and they do not show surface expression of the mu chain at this stage (Figure 5-1). Pre-B cells already have selected the variable region that will be part of the immunoglobulin heavy chain which their plasma cell progeny will eventually produce. Pre-B cells divide at a rapid rate (generation time is about 12 hours), leading to the production of small pre-B lymphocytes that still contain cytoplasmic mu. At this stage allelic exclusion occurs wherein either the kappa or lambda gene is selected for production. Although there will be subsequent shifts of the heavy chain expression, the light chain remains constant for this clone. On the surface of the cell, one finds CALLA, Ia, B1, B2, and B4.

The next stage of development is called an immature B lymphocyte. In the fetus, these cells can be recognized by the tenth to twelfth week of gestation

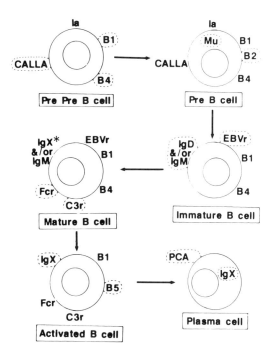

Figure 5-1. B-cell maturation. Markers outlined at different stages indicate the earliest stage at which those markers are usually detected.

[8]. They contain surface whole IgM molecules with the selected light chain. At this stage of development, the variable regions of both the light and heavy chain will be the same as those in the immunoglobulins produced by the plasma cell progeny of these immature B cells. Although IgM is the major surface isotype at this stage, it will usually not be the ultimate isotype produced by this clone. These immature B lymphocytes are most easily tolerized by presenting antigens at this stage of development. The immature B cells also acquire receptors for the Epstein-Barr virus (EBVr). They continue to express antigens marked by the monoclonal antibodies B1 and B4.

As these cells develop into mature B lymphocytes, they contain surface IgM, often together with surface IgD (Figure 5-1). The variable region portion of the IgD is the same as that of the IgM, and the light chain of both immunoglobulins is the same. The genes for the heavy chain will usually change as the B lymphocytes mature to plasma cells and, at times, express more than one isotype, while the light chain is always the same; understanding this helps one to understand the occurrence of so-called biclonal gammopathies. In most biclonal gammopathies, both M proteins have the same light chain type. When the light chains are the same, it is likely that we are seeing expression of two heavy chain genes in the same clone. This merely recapitulates the events seen during development. When the light chain types differ, however, the M components truly arise from different clones. The mature B cells also develop receptors for the Fc portion of IgG (Fcr) and for C3 (C3r).

After the B lymphocytes are activated by combination with antigen with the appropriate costimulation by macrophages and helper T cells, they become activated B cells. These cells acquire a receptor for B5 and may lose the EBVr. Thereafter, the B cells mature to plasma cells. These cells synthesize and secrete large amounts of the immunoglobulin; however, they do not express the immunoglobulin on the surface as do the B lymphocytes. They do express an antigen marked by the monoclonal antibody PCA-1.

T-LYMPHOCYTE DEVELOPMENT

Although the detection of T-cell dysfunctions is not a major subject for a book on serum protein electrophoresis, their intimate interactions with B lymphocytes and the alterations in the resulting plasma cell products are relevant for this chapter.

Like B cells, T lymphocytes must mature through successive stages of development. Stem cells in the bone marrow give rise to cells that are precommitted to become T cells. These migrate to the thymus gland where, under the influence of thymic factors, they proliferate and acquire cell-surface receptors characteristic of T lymphocytes. Originally, T lymphocytes were recognized by the presence of a receptor for sheep erythrocytes. A rosette assay was convenient because it allowed one to stain the rosetted cells and determine if the T-cell population was indeed anaplastic. Recently, with the development of monoclonal antibody technology and flow cytometry techniques, many markers are available to define different subpopulations of T lymphocytes [10].

The production of new monoclonal antibodies to T- and B-cell surface molecules is almost too rapid to be appreciated. However, there are a few major monoclonal antibodies that help us to understand maturation of T lymphocytes. One scheme, from the work of Reinherz et al. [11], has proven particularly useful (Figure 5–2). Early on in the thymus, these cells (termed thymocytes at this stage of development) acquire two antigens, which react with the monoclonal antibodies T11 (OK-T11, Ortho) and Leu 9 (Bectin-Dickinson). Studies have shown that anti-T11 reacts with (or close to) the receptor for sheep erythrocytes discussed above. Leu 9 appears somewhat earlier than T11, which is a good marker for the total T-cell population. Early in thymic development the cells acquire receptors for T10 and T9, although these antibodies are not specific for T cells (they can react with other leukocytes).

Later, at the common thymocyte stage, cells express both T4 and T8 receptors. As cells mature to the late thymocyte stage two major events can be recognized. First, cells acquire a marker for relative maturity and function

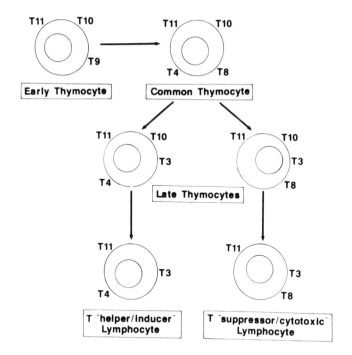

Figure 5-2.   T-cell maturation.

(T3, a structure associated with the antigen receptor), and cells express only T4 or T8, not both. Finally, cells leave the thymus to become T lymphocytes in peripheral blood. At this stage they lose the T10 marker.

The functions of some of these populations are known. T lymphocytes that bear T4 are said to be the "helper/inducer" population, while those that bear T8 are said to be the "suppressor/cytotoxic" population. While this is true in general, it is important to be aware that these statements are vast over-simplifications of what is really known about the individual cells in those populations. Specifically, it is known that when T4 cells are purified and placed in tissue culture with B lymphocytes, they will "help" those B lymphocytes mature into plasma cells. However, it is also clear that only a minority (perhaps less than 10%) of those T4 cells are actually providing the help. The function of the majority of cells in that population is not known.

Therefore, an increase in the number of T4 cells in peripheral blood may correlate with the presence of an increased immunoglobulin production. However, if the particular T4, or T8, cells that have proliferated are not the specific ones capable of "helping" B-cell responses, no such helper effect will be seen. When interpreting T- and B-cell marker data, it is useful to remember these limitations.

CONDITIONS ASSOCIATED
WITH MONOCLONAL GAMMOPATHIES

With electrophoretic techniques having less resolution than those described in this volume, only relatively large monoclonal gammopathies could be detected with confidence. Therefore, aside from multiple myeloma and Waldenstrom's macroglobulinemia, in samples studied using the five-band serum protein electrophoresis pattern it was difficult to detect small gammopathies unless one also performed immunoelectrophoresis. Even then, gammopathies readily evident with HRE were often not detected. The current clinical literature on serum protein electrophoresis and the incidence of monoclonal gammopathies in B-cell neoplasms lags far behind the technical capabilities for the detection of these gammopathies.

We define a monoclonal gammopathy as the electrophoretically and antigenically homogeneous protein product of a single clone of maturing B lymphocytes and/or plasma cells that has proliferated beyond the constraints of normal control mechanisms. The monoclonal protein may be found in the serum and/or urine, depending on its size and the renal function. A wide variety of conditions has been associated with such monoclonal proliferations (Table 5-1). At one end of the spectrum is multiple myeloma; at the other end is monoclonal gammopathy of undetermined significance (MGUS). Despite its clumsiness, the latter term accurately denotes the fact that we are occasionally unsure as to the relevance of a gammopathy for a particular patient.

It should not be surprising that such a broad spectrum of disease exists in patients with plasma cell neoplasms (which is what the presence of a monoclonal gammopathy implies). A neoplasm is not equivalent to a malignancy, and the situation with B-cell/plasma-cell neoplasms parallels the more familiar proliferations of other cell types. For instance, a similar spectrum of behavior is seen in neoplastic proliferations of squamous epithelium. Dysplasia of the cervix is graded from mild to severe or *in situ* carcinoma; squamous cell carcinoma of the cervix may be microinvasive or may invade and metastasize. Mild dysplasia does not necessarily progress to carcinoma; however, since it has propensity to do so, it needs to be followed carefully. These features parallel the situation in B-lymphocyte/plasma-cell neoplasms, in which detecting and characterizing a monoclonal gammopathy provides information about a neoplastic process that must be immediately studied, to determine its position in the spectrum, and then either treated or followed at a regular interval (depending on the specific diagnosis).

First, we review specific clinical situations and the use of HRE, immunofixation, immunoglobulin quantification (including kappa and lambda measurements), and immunoelectrophoresis (IEP) (on concentrated urine) to establish the presence of the monoclonal gammopathies. Second, we detail our laboratory strategy for specimens to diagnose monoclonal gammopathy in 1 day (for most patients) and to eliminate expensive needless testing when not indicated.

Table 5-1 Classification of Monoclonal Gammopathies

			Most Frequent HRE Picture
I.	Multiple myeloma		
	Immunoglobulin		
		IgG	Large gamma spike
		IgM	Broad spike at origin
		IgA	Broad beta spike
		IgD	Small gamma or beta spike
		IgE	Small beta spike
		Light chain disease	Low gamma, occasional
		(kappa, lambda)	small spike (beta)
		Heavy Chain Disease	Broad beta band
		(alpha, mu, gamma)	
		Biclonal gammopathy	Two gamma spikes
		Nonsecretory	Normal or low gamma
II.	Waldenstrom's macroglobulinemia		
		IgM	Broad band near origin
		IgA	Broad band near origin
		IgG	Broad band near origin
III.	B-Lymphocyte neoplasms		
		Chronic lymphocytic leukemia	Low gamma, small band
		Well-differentiated lymphocytic	Low gamma, small band
IV.	Amyloid		
		With multiple myeloma	Gamma spike
		Not associated with myeloma	Normal, low gamma
V.	Monoclonal gammopathy occasionally associated with other clinical conditions		
	Autoimmune disease		
		Rheumatoid arthritis	
		Systemic lupus erythematosus	
		Polymyositis	
		Cold agglutinin disease	
	Peripheral neuropathy		
	Epithelial neoplasms		
VI.	Monoclonal gammopathy of undetermined significance (MGUS)		

Multiple Myeloma

Multiple myeloma is a malignant neoplasm of plasma cells (although earlier stages of neoplastic B lymphocytes may be found) that usually presents with bone marrow involvement. Typically, these cells synthesize and secrete considerable amounts of monoclonal whole immunoglobulin and/or monoclonal free light chains (Bence Jones protein). The prominent bone marrow involvement in this disease is associated with lytic lesions in the ribs, vertebrae, skull, and long bones along with bone pain and pathologic fractures.

As discussed earlier, plasma cells are at the terminal stage of B-lymphocyte differentiation and as such they usually lack surface immunoglobulin. Similarly, neoplastic plasma cells in multiple myeloma lack surface immunoglobulins despite the copious secretions they produce [12,13]. Those few myeloma cells that do demonstrate surface immunoglobulin also often bear the B-cell marker B1 (Figure 5-1), indicating they may be at a more immature stage of development than normal plasma cells. A histologic correlate of this immaturity and malignant behavior is the large atypical cells that may be seen, occasionally with binucleate cells in the involved marrow. However, the criteria of atypical nuclei and multinucleate plasma cells are insufficient to absolutely distinguish between proliferating polyclonal plasma cells in (for instance) chronic osteomyelitis and monoclonal plasma cells of multiple myeloma. Such an exercise is fortunately unnecessary because the electrophoretic or (in the case of nonsecretory myeloma) immunohistologic techniques described later in this chapter provide definitive information for this differentiation.

Although multiple myeloma is mainly a disease of malignant plasma cells, there is good evidence that in patients with myeloma both circulating B lymphocytes and even pre-B cells in the bone marrow can be found that express the specific idiotype of the monoclonal protein being produced by the myeloma cells from that patient [14–16]. The finding of such precursor cells may seem surprising considering that the neoplasm is characterized by mature-appearing plasma cells. However, this is entirely consistent with our understanding of the variable maturation in neoplastic cells. For instance, a squamous cell carcinoma may consist mainly of mature keratinized cells, yet one is not at all surprised to find some immature nonkeratinizing elements in the same neoplasm.

At one time, myeloma protein products were thought to be "abnormal" molecules, hence the term paraproteinemia or dysproteinemia. Although occasional monoclonal gammopathies have deletions or other unusual characteristics, it is now clear that most monoclonal immunoglobulins represent massive overproduction of molecules, each of which is structurally normal. Indeed, the antigen-binding capability of several monoclonal proteins has been determined, and some occur with surprising frequency.

The prevalence of monoclonal gammopathies of the major immunoglobulin isotypes roughly parallels the concentration of that immunoglobulin in serum. For instance, in his large series of patients with myeloma, Kyle [17] found an IgG monoclonal protein in about 60% of cases while an IgA myeloma only occurred in about 25%, and that kappa light chain disease is twice as frequent as lambda (consistent with the normal 2:1 ratio of kappa to lambda in the serum). All IgM cases were considered as a separate category under Waldenstrom's in this series.

There are, however, some notable exceptions to this generalization. Among the subclasses of IgG, Schur et al. [18] found significantly fewer cases of IgG2 than would be predicted by its concentration in the serum. Similar observations have been made about the infrequence of IgA2 monoclonal gammopathies [18,19].

Immunoglobulin Isotypes

In most cases of myeloma, electrophoretic findings are straightforward. The characteristic densely staining spike typically occurs in the gamma region, near the origin, and in the beta region for IgG, IgM, and IgA monoclonal proteins, respectively (Figure 5-3). IgG myeloma proteins are almost always 7 S, 160,000-dalton monomers that only rarely produce problems with hyperviscosity. IgA gammopathies can occur as monomers or as polymers with variable molecular weight. As these molecules can self-aggregate, they have been known to cause problems with hyperviscosity. Since most of the IgA monoclonal gammopathies migrate in the beta region, they may be masked by the C3 and transferrin bands on serum protein electrophoresis. Furthermore, plasma would have a large fibrinogen band in the exact location of the monoclonal IgA gammopathy shown in Figure 5-3. This is one of the reasons to quantify IgG, IgA, and IgM as well as kappa- and lambda-containing immunoglobulins to rule out a monoclonal process. Although unusual, IgM may be the main

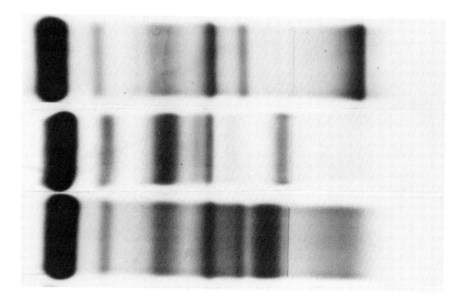

Figure 5-3. Three samples with monoclonal proteins in typical positions for their heavy chain class. Top sample has an IgG monoclonal protein migrating in the mid-gamma region. Middle sample has an IgM monoclonal protein near the origin. Bottom sample has a broad IgA monoclonal protein just cathodal to the C3 band. Although these are typical locations for monoclonal proteins of these isotypes, they may migrate at a variety of locations from alpha-2 to the slow gamma.

immunoglobulin in cases of multiple myeloma, accounting for about 1% of cases. IgM myeloma is associated with plasma cell proliferations as opposed to the more typical IgM monoclonal gammopathies (part of Waldenstrom's macroglobulinemia) in which lymphoplasmacytoid cells are seen [20,21].

IgD myelomas are uncommon, accounting for only 2% of cases, but they have some characteristics of which one must be aware to avoid misdiagnosis. The kappa/lambda ratio for the reported cases is 1:9. Even with the older five-band electrophoretic technique, almost 90% of patients were reported to have "M components." While these are usually in the gamma region, 25% of cases have beta spikes, and in one case the monoclonal component was in the alpha-2 region [22]. IgD myeloma may be missed because the M components can be relatively small, and studies using the five-band electrophoretic techniques noted that the M component may be hidden by the normal alpha-2 or beta proteins. Further, when quantification is performed by radial immunodiffusion, at least two dilutions of the patient's serum must be used to avoid the possibility of antigen excess, which may result in a false-negative for IgD; this is the only situation in which quantification of IgD is indicated [23]. IgD myeloma should always be suspected when a light chain is identified in the serum by immunofixation or immunoelectrophoresis but there is no corresponding heavy chain (gamma, mu, or alpha). While suspicion should be greater for lambda than for kappa spikes, the latter do occur with IgD monoclonal gammopathies. Patients with IgD myeloma more frequently have Bence Jones proteinuria than do patients with other heavy chain types, and extraosseous spread is common. Cytoplasmic crystalline inclusions and amyloid have been described in patients with IgD myeloma [24,25]. The latter sometimes require immunohistochemical identification (discussed later).

IgE myeloma is rare. The few reported patients have been younger than is typical for myeloma, and the disease pursues a relatively rapid course. This seems somewhat paradoxical; although some patients present with plasma cell leukemia, most do not have either osteolytic bone lesions or hypercalcemia, although they do have increased osteosclerosis, and hyperviscosity has been described [26,27]. As with IgD myelomas, finding a light chain in the serum without a corresponding heavy chain should provoke the laboratory to quantify the serum for IgD and IgE. If IgE is present at elevated concentrations, immunofixation should be performed to identify the monoclonality.

Light Chain Disease

Monoclonal light chains (Bence Jones protein) often accompany intact monoclonal proteins, and are the only element of monoclonal proteins in patients with light chain disease. Plasma cells are often viewed as though they were efficiently producing intact molecules consisting of two heavy and two light chains (Chapter 2). In fact, even some normal plasma cells are more like poorly organized factories producing too many light chains for the number of heavy chains available. The excess free light chains are secreted from the cell along with intact immunoglobulins. The small size of the light chains allows them to pass through the glomerular basement membrane into the glomerular filtrate, from which they are reabsorbed by the proximal convoluted tubules. In myeloma, when large amounts of the free monoclonal light chains are present, they overwhelm the capacity of the proximal convoluted tubules and can be detected in the urine. It is important to note that conditions associated with polyclonal plasma cell expansion can also produce excessive free light chains, which may be detected in the urine. However, such chains are polyclonal and are not Bence Jones protein (BJP). It is important to separate polyclonal free light chains from monoclonal free light chains for diagnostic purposes; only the latter are BJP. The presence of BJP in urine samples often portends a poorer prognosis, as this protein is much more frequently seen in association with myeloma (50–60%) and amyloidosis (60%) than it is with "benign monoclonal gammopathy" (14%) [28,29].

Bence Jones proteins occur in several forms. When they are secreted by the plasma cells as monomers or dimers with molecular weights of 22,000–44,000, it is unusual to see a large serum spike. Rather, the protein passes into the urine where it can be detected by electrophoresis on concentrated urine (Figure 5–4). We concentrate an early-morning urine sample for 4 hours, using the Amicon miniconcentrators, which is usually 100-fold for urine without proteinuria and often considerably less (about 20-fold) for urine with heavy protein. However, as electrophoresis alone is not sensitive enough to detect all BJP, we characterize all urine samples suspected of having BJP by IEP (Figure 5–5).

Although only a handful of patients with tetrameric light chain disease have been reported, Solling et al. [30] found that 25% of patients with kappa-secreting myelomas have detectable tetrameric kappa chains in their serum (usually coexisting with dimeric and monomeric forms). The reported cases of tetrameric light chain disease are dramatic because BJP is *only* in the serum and not in the urine, which often sends the laboratorian off on a fruitless effort to identify the nonexistent heavy chain. However, aside from this in-

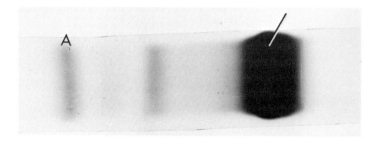

Figure 5–4.   HRE of urine shows an enormous gamma band (*indicated*). The albumin band (A) is quite small.

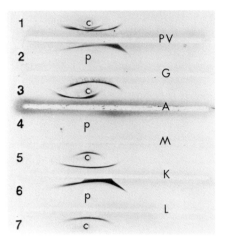

Figure 5-5. IEP of sample shown in Figure 5-4 shows a large kappa Bence Jones protein that extends into the trough in both the polyvalent and antikappa reaction. Symbols: c, control (serum); p, patient urine; PV, polyvalent; G, anti-IgG; A, anti-IgA; M, anti-IgM; K, kappa; L, lambda.

terest, the evidence suggests that polymerization of light chains does not increase the nephrotoxicity of BJP [30]. Some experimental studies have suggested a relationship between the isoelectric point (pI; see Chapter 1) of BJP and renal damage. Lambda monoclonal proteins with a pI > 5.7 elicited greater renal damage than those with a lower pI when given to experimental animals [31]. Others have found that abnormal molecular structure, size or glycosylation may explain the variation in nephrotoxicity that occurs from case to case [32]. It is important to note that patients do not need to have multiple myeloma to sustain renal damage with BJP.

Several groups have reported that patients with lambda light chain disease do significantly poorer than those with kappa light chain disease, although the cause for this difference is unknown [33]. There does not seem to be any difference in the extent of renal involvement, degree of anemia, number of osteolytic lesions, or incidence of amyloidosis between the two light chain types [34]. When BJP are reabsorbed by the tubules, they may damage the nephron, and an acquired adult Fanconi's syndrome can result. These patients can have a paradoxically low serum calcium due to loss from the urine [35].

In diagnosing light chain disease, it is important to discard the use of the classic heat precipitation test of the urine. Most BJP that are in the urine in large quantities will precipitate when heated to 56°C and upon further heating will dissolve; unfortunately, so will some polymeric light chains. Further, the heat test misses at least 30–50% of true monoclonal free light chains, because some BJP will not behave in this fashion at any concentration and others are present in too small an amount to be detected by this insensitive method [36]. HRE on urine concentrated 100 times will typically show multiple bands as these molecules tend to polymerize forming monomers, dimers and tetramers (Figure 5-6). However, IEP of such urine usually shows only a single band (Figure 5-7).

Lambda light chains occur preferentially as dimers, whereas kappa light chains occur in a variety of forms. Although most of the monomeric and dimeric forms of light chains are quickly excreted into the urine, the sensitivity of immunofixation can allow their detection in the serum (Figure 5-8). Obviously, because of the size of tetramers, these are found mainly in the serum,

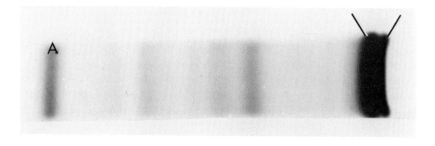

Figure 5-6. HRE of urine shows a double, show gamma band (*indicated*). Albumin (A) is relatively faint.

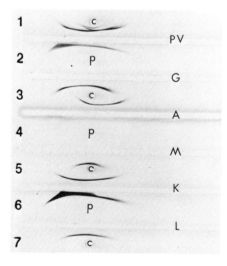

Figure 5-7. IEP of urine sample shown in Figure 5-6 shows a single kappa Bence Jones protein that extends into the troughs of both the polyvalent and antikappa reaction. (Symbols as in Figure 5-5.)

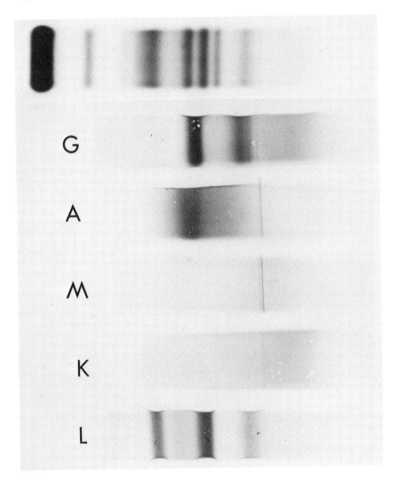

Figure 5–8.   This serum has a complex HRE and immunofixation pattern. There are three bands in the beta region of the HRE strip instead of the usual two, and just anodal to the origin another faint band can be seen. The immunofixation pattern shows two discrete bands in the IgG reaction, accounting for the two bands described above. The IgA reaction shows a diffuse pattern with some restricted mobility in the fast beta area. The lack of a light chain in this region indicates that the IgA is polyclonal. In the lambda reaction, three bands are noted, of which two correspond exactly to the IgG bands. This would be consistent with either an IgG lambda biclonal gammopathy or with self-aggregation of some of the IgG lambda (explaining its slight migration out of the origin). Also, there is a third anodal band in the lambda reaction with no corresponding heavy chain; this is free lambda light chain, which was also found in this patient's urine.

unless considerable renal damage has occurred. By HRE alone, other proteins such as hemoglobin, myoglobin, or lysozyme may be confused with BJP. Therefore, in patients suspected of having light chain disease, IEP of concentrated urine (100-fold) should be performed. Immunofixation may be used, but because of the lack of standard methods to quantify kappa- and lambda-containing immunoglobulins in the urine, extreme antigen or antibody excess may occur (Chapter 4) and a BJP may be missed.

While most cases with BJP give a characteristic pattern, interpretation of urine IEP can be difficult. Usually there is a marked difference between the quantity of kappa and lambda, with the BJP giving a strong precipitation arc and often spilling into the reagent antibody trough (Figures 5-5 and 5-7). In cases with small amounts of BJP the difference between the kappa and the lambda arcs can be quite subtle. Furthermore, some patients with polyclonal increases in light chain can have both kappa and lambda, which even experienced observers have overcalled when the proportion was not exactly 2:1 (Figure 5-9). When the urine is not sufficiently concentrated or when relatively little immunoglobulin is passing into the urine, a small kappa arc with no lambda arc may be seen (Figure 5-10). This also has been misdiagnosed as BJP. By performing both HRE and IEP on these samples, one can improve diagnostic accuracy. The HRE will show the restricted mobility (often in multiple bands reflecting polymerization) while the IEP will demonstrate the light chain type. Ideally, quantification of kappa and lambda chains followed by immunofixation at the appropriate dilution should be performed. At this time, however, techniques to quantify kappa and lambda in the urine are not well standardized.

Bence Jones proteins are seen in the serum in three circumstances. When they occur as tetrameric light chains they are too large to pass through the glomerular basement membrane and usually produce a spike in the serum. A second and common cause of BJP in the serum is as a result of renal damage with sufficient loss of nephrons to reduce the clearance of these and other molecules. Third, BJP may bind to other serum proteins including prealbumin, albumin, alpha-1 antitrypsin, and transferrin (Figure 5-11) [36,37]. The latter can usually be demonstrated by finding numerous bands by immunofixation that resolve upon treatment with 2-mercaptoethanol. Nonetheless, when a monoclonal light chain is identified in the serum, it is incumbent on the laboratorian to rule out the possibility of IgD or IgE myeloma.

Nonsecretory Myeloma

Nonsecretory myeloma is reported to occur in about 1% of patients with multiple myeloma. These are cases of monoclonal plasma cell proliferations in which no monoclonal protein can be detected in the serum or urine by conventional electrophoretic techniques. To be thorough, one should rule out cryoglobulins, which may result in a false-negative electrophoretic study. Clinically, nonsecretory myelomas behave similarly to other cases of multiple mye-

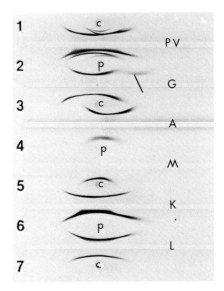

Figure 5-9.   Urine IEP shows several precipitin lines with polyvalent reagent. One goes into the trough. With the anti-IgG reagent, a gullwing pattern is seen. The densely staining area is IgG whole molecule, and the indicated faintly staining area is Fc fragment (from IgG broken down in the urine). There is a faint IgA precipitin band, and no reaction of the patient's urine occurred with anti-IgM. There are large precipitin bands in both the kappa and lambda reaction. Because the kappa reaction proceeded well into the trough, this sample was erroneously called a kappa Bence Jones protein, which it is not. The normal kappa/lambda ratio is about 2:1 and that is roughly what is seen here. Be sure to correlate the HRE pattern of the urine with the IEP. When there is enough monoclonal light chain to cause the reaction to go into the trough, a large dense area of restricted mobility should be seen on the HRE pattern. (Symbols as in Figure 5-5.)

loma, and it is not known why these plasma cells fail to secrete a detectable product. Various studies have shown failure to secrete, or rapid degradation of, an abnormal immunoglobulin product. In fact, studies by Alanen et al. [38] indicated that Mott cells (plasma cells with large intracytoplasmic inclusions of immunoglobulin) have a partial or complete block of the secretion of these molecules. The plasma cells in this condition clearly contain a monoclonal immunoglobulin, which is best detected by immunohistochemical analysis [39].

We have found that intracytoplasmic immunoglobulin can be detected conveniently on routine formalin-fixed paraffin-embedded tissues. Tissue sections are cut at 4 μm and mounted on glass slides coated with Sobo glue (Sloman's, Inc.), which prevents detachment during subsequent steps but does not interfere with fluorescence. The tissue sections are then deparaffinized with

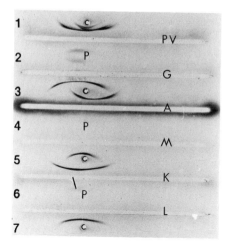

Figure 5-10. This urine IEP has very little immunoglobulin protein. As seen in the polyvalent reaction, only a tiny arc is present near the origin. The same arc is seen in the IgG reaction, indicating that virtually all the immunoglobulin present is intact IgG. The kappa and the lambda reactions show only a small amount of kappa with no lambda detectable. This is not an IgG kappa monoclonal protein. There is just too little lambda present for the reaction to be seen by IEP. (Symbols as in Figure 5-5.)

xylene and brought back through serial dilutions of alcohol to a water rinse. Next, the sections are digested with a solution of 50 mg trypsin with 50 mg CaCl$_2$ in 50 ml of water adjusted to pH 7.8. Following digestion at 37°C for 2 hours, the slides are washed and then stained with fluorescein-conjugated anti-human kappa and rhodamine-conjugated anti-human lambda chain. This double staining technique is helpful in preventing overinterpretation. Because some preparations are poorly fixed, some cells nonspecifically absorb serum kappa and lambda. These would then react with the conjugates and may be erroneously read as positive. With the present technique, when a cell stains with both the antikappa and antilambda reagents it would fluoresce both green and red and we would know that some artifact is occurring. (I call this "immunogarbage.") But the most important thing is to avoid using cells that stain in that manner for diagnosis. As in the case shown in Figures 5-12 and 5-13, the monoclonality is usually obvious [40].

Heavy Chain Disease

Heavy chain disease is extremely uncommon, especially in the Western world. The most frequent form is alpha heavy chain disease, which occurs mainly in the Middle East and Mediterranean region [41]. The tissue distribution of alpha heavy chain disease roughly parallels that of the normal distribution of IgA along the gut and bronchial mucosa, but it has been reported in other

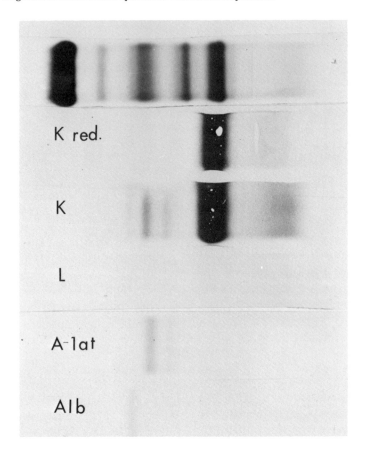

Figure 5-11. This serum has a densely staining band in the C3 area. When immunofixation was performed with antikappa (K) and antilambda (L), the dense kappa band was seen indicating that this was a kappa monoclonal protein. No reaction was seen with the other heavy chain antisera (not shown). Also in the kappa reaction were three other bands. When the serum was reduced with 2-mercaptoethanol (K red.), these extra bands disappeared. They were identified by performing immunofixation of the purified kappa chain with antisera to alpha-1 antitrypsin (A-1at) and albumin (Alb).

locations [42]. Clinically, the patients usually have slow progression of their disease during the early phase, and, importantly, cures have been reported when treatment was received at this stage [43].

Unlike typical multiple myeloma, alpha heavy chain disease is usually difficult to diagnose in the clinical laboratory because serum protein electrophoresis and IEP often fail to disclose the presence of the monoclonal protein. Since there is no monoclonal light chain, the disease must be established by demonstrating the lack of light chain in the presence of excessive heavy alpha chains. An immunoselection technique has been used to assist in this diag-

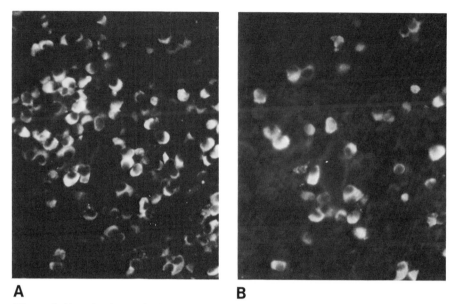

Figure 5–12. A. Control plasma cells stained with fluorescein antikappa. B. Same field as A but stained with rhodamine antilambda. This is a polyclonal pattern.

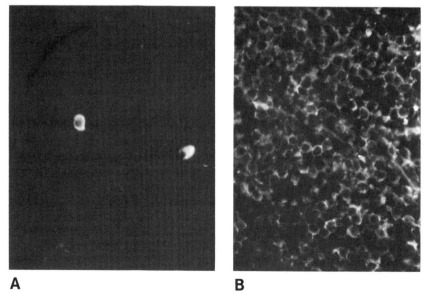

Figure 5–13. A. Patient plasma cells stained with fluorescein antikappa. Only two cells are positive. B. Same field as A, but stained with rhodamine antilambda. This is a monoclonal lymphoplasmacytic infiltrate due to the marked predominance of the lambda-containing cells. Note that the lambda-containing cells had less cytoplasm, indicating that they were at an earlier stage of maturation than plasma cells.

nosis. For this, antikappa and antilambda antisera are mixed into the agarose (as is done for radial immunodiffusion) and standard IEP is carried out. Since intact immunoglobulin molecules contain either kappa or lambda chains, they will precipitate around the sample well; the distance from the well roughly correlates with concentration. However, the alpha chains will form a beta-migrating precipitin arc with the antialpha antisera [44].

By serum protein electrophoresis, the heavy chain diseases display non-specific patterns. For alpha chain disease, a broad beta band is the most typical, although more discrete bands and gamma-migrating bands have been reported [45]. Similarly, the electrophoretic pattern of gamma heavy chain disease is nonspecific, giving a relatively broad band anywhere from the alpha-2 through the gamma region. Kyle [17] cautioned against being too complacent when seeing such a band. Whereas alpha chain disease usually has symptoms relating to the mucosal surfaces, gamma heavy chain disease (Franklin's disease) has systemic symptoms more reminiscent of lymphoma: generalized lymphadenopathy, hepatosplenomegaly, pleural effusions, and ascites. In addition, there is often edema of the uvula and soft palate. Histological examination will demonstrate infiltrates in the involved tissues with atypical lymphocytes and plasma cells [46–48]. Mu heavy chain disease is extremely rare, but has shown the same picture as gamma chain disease [49].

Biclonal Gammopathies

Biclonal gammopathies (or double gammopathies, as we prefer) are uncommon and can be somewhat confusing. It is important to understand this condition, because two monoclonal gammopathies in the same serum are being detected more frequently with HRE than was possible with older five-band electrophoretic systems. The term "biclonal" implies that the plasma cell neoplasm arose from two separate clones of B lymphocytes. As such, they should always have a different variable region (idiotype) and may differ in light chain class. It is not reasonable to attempt to distinguish between two different idiotypes in clinical laboratories. The presence of different light chains is *a priori* evidence that the neoplasm represents the product of two separate clones, which would be true "biclonal" gammopathies. However, most reported cases and most we have seen in our laboratory have had the same light chain type with two different heavy or heavy chain subclass types (Figure 5-14). The vast majority of these cases really represent one clone of B-lymphocyte progeny that is expressing two different heavy chain constant regions (similar to the stage in B-cell ontogeny where both IgM and another heavy chain class are present on the surface of the B cell) (Figure 5-1). Therefore, for cases with the same light chain type we prefer the term "double gammopathy," which recognizes the fact that two distinct proteins are seen but does not imply that they resulted from two separate clones.

Double gammopathies constitute about 5% of patients with monoclonal gammopathies [17,50,51]. Some heavy chain classes occur more frequently in

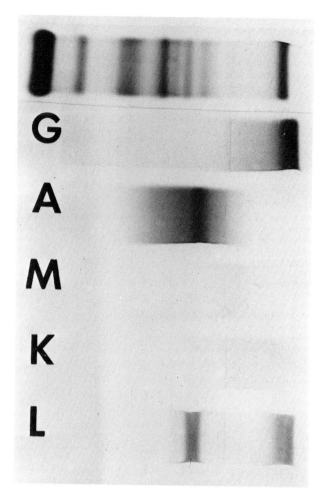

Figure 5-14. HRE shows two unusual bands. The gamma band is obvious, and a weak beta band is also seen in the fibrinogen area. The irregular band between transferrin and C3 is beta-1 lipoprotein. Immunofixation revealed that the two bands represent a double gammopathy, IgG lambda and IgA lambda. (Symbols as in earlier figures.)

double gammopathies with IgG-IgM occurring most frequently followed by IgG-IgA, IgG-IgG (detected by their different electrophoretic mobilities), and IgA-IgM [52].

The reasons for the occurrence of double gammopathies are better understood by examining the structure of the immunoglobulin heavy chain constant-region gene sequence (Figure 5-15). When a cell switches from one heavy chain class to another, such as from mu to gamma 3, the intervening

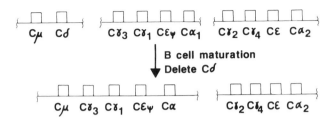

Figure 5-15. Schematic representation of heavy chain gene rearrangement during B-cell maturation. While intervening genes are deleted (such as delta in this case) during maturation of a particular clone, the remaining heavy chain genes are still available and may be selected for expression at a later time in maturation. This could result in the double gammopathies; that is, two heavy chains that originated from a single clone.

genes (in this case delta) are deleted and cannot be expressed later [53]. The remaining segments, however, could be selected and subsequently expressed. This occurs normally during B-lymphocyte maturation where B cells often bear both surface IgM and another heavy chain isotype (Figure 5-1). Hammarstrom et al. [19] recently reported that in gammopathies with two heavy chain classes but only one light chain type (double gammopathies), there may be preferential switches to explain the frequency of the two heavy chain types observed. There is no known clinical significance to the demonstration of double (or even true biclonal) gammopathies. Most of these patients have "monoclonal gammopathy of undetermined significance" (see later discussion), while others have B-cell lymphoproliferative disorders or multiple myeloma.

Hypogammaglobulinemia in Myeloma

In multiple myeloma, concomitant suppression of the normal immunoglobulin secretion is a key feature recognized by examining the electrophoretic pattern (Figure 5-16). Although this deficiency has been known for many years and correlates with an increased susceptibility to infectious diseases, it is still unclear why it occurs. From our earlier review of B-cell ontogeny, one might assume that a problem with normal B-cell maturation may occur in myeloma patients. *In vitro* studies have confirmed that peripheral blood lymphocytes from patients with multiple myeloma have a poor response to B-cell mitogens [54]. These data are also consistent with recent studies that there is a profound decrease (as much as 20- to 600-fold in the normal polyclonal B lymphocytes) in the circulation of patients with multiple myeloma, implying the existence of a suppressive influence on B-lymphocyte maturation. Interestingly, the number of B cells does not seem to correlate with disease status or the concentration of the monoclonal protein [55].

The decrease in normal immunoglobulins that occurs in myeloma patients likely relates to excessive suppressor-T-cell activities and deficient helper-

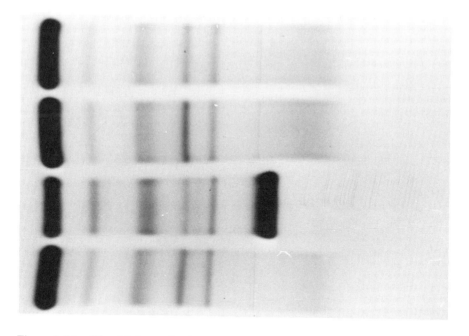

Figure 5-16. The third sample, from a patient with myeloma, shows a large monoclonal spike at the origin. Note that the gamma globulin area has very little of the normal hazy staining seen in the samples above and below. This is caused by suppression of normal immunoglobulin production in myeloma.

T-cell numbers and function [56–58]. It is clear that the T-cell populations can influence polyclonal immunoglobulin production and B-cell development. Patients with helper-T-cell lymphomas often have a polyclonal increase in gamma globulin [59]. One must be careful to avoid oversimplification. For instance, most of the helper T cells of patients with the acquired immune deficiency syndrome (AIDS) have been destroyed by infection with the HTLV-III virus, yet a polyclonal increase in gamma globulin is consistently found in their serum. The cause of the altered T-lymphocyte function in myeloma patients remains unknown. Some experimental studies have suggested that the production of an RNA-containing plasma factor might influence the immunoglobulin production [60,61]. But the nature of such a factor and its specific effects on the immune system remain to be defined.

Waldenstrom's Macroglobulinemia

Waldenstrom's macroglobulinemia differs from multiple myeloma in several clinical aspects. Patients with this disease do not have lytic skeletal lesions, and usually present with fatigue and weakness due to anemia and hyperviscosity. They usually have an increased bleeding tendency, often resulting in epistaxis and cutaneous purpuric lesions. Hyperviscosity is a key feature of this disease, which produces significant neurologic complaints, cardiac insufficiency, and resultant vascular insufficiency throughout the body. IgM is by far the major immunoglobulin class associated with this condition. Indeed, some authorities will claim that when a monoclonal IgM is present the disease *is* Waldenstrom's macroglobulinemia, but this seems to be an unwarranted oversimplification. IgG, IgA, and IgE monoclonal proteins that behave clinically like Waldenstrom's have been described from some patients, and these deserve to be classified by the clinical picture rather than the heavy chain isotype [62]. Further, it is also clear that some patients with IgM monoclonal proteins have the clinical picture of multiple myeloma, including lytic skeletal lesions, and should be treated accordingly [21].

The clinical course of Waldenstrom's macroglobulinemia is slow relative to that in multiple myeloma, although exceptional cases have been noted [63]. Hyperviscosity usually causes significant clinical problems when the IgM level is greater than 2000 mg/dl [17]. Histologically, the bone marrow is infiltrated with lymphoplasmacytoid cells, the monoclonality of which can be demonstrated by the immunohistologic technique described earlier in this chapter. Uncommonly, cases of Waldenstrom's macroglobulinemia will evolve into an immunoblastic sarcoma. Leonhard et al. [64] noted that a decrease in the concentration of the monoclonal IgM may herald the progression to a more malignant, hence less differentiated, cell type.

On serum protein electrophoresis, the typical case of Waldenstrom's macroglobulinemia shows an M component either at the origin or just anodal or cathodal to it (Figure 5-17). This electrophoretic behavior reflects both the isoelectric point of IgM and that it is usually a pentamer with a molecular

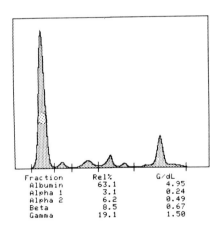

Fraction	Rel%	G/dL
Albumin	63.1	4.95
Alpha 1	3.1	0.24
Alpha 2	6.2	0.49
Beta	8.5	0.67
Gamma	19.1	1.50

Figure 5-17. Densitometric scan of serum showing a spike near the origin.

weight of around 1,000,000 that will often self-aggregate. Immunoglobulin quantification usually demonstrates a severalfold increase of IgM, while IgG and IgA are typically in the normal range. Despite the rather obvious M component on HRE and considerable increase in IgM, due to the umbrella effect (Chapter 4), it may not be possible to determine the monoclonality of the lesion by IEP although the result is obvious by immunofixation (Figure 5-18).

There are several possible solutions to the problem of the umbrella effect. In many cases, by treating the monoclonal IgM with 2-mercaptoethanol, the intermonomer disulfide bonds will be cleaved and the monoclonal component can be determined by repeat IEP [65]. Also, the serum can be placed on a Sephadex G-200 molecular sieving column or its equivalent. The larger molecules, which elute first from the column, can be concentrated and rerun

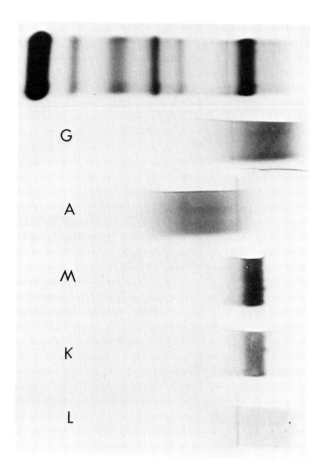

Figure 5-18. Immunofixation of serum shown in Figure 5-17 indicates that the restriction is due to an IgM kappa monoclonal protein. (Symbols as in Figure 5-5.)

on IEP for the diagnosis. Available commercial diethylaminoethyl cellulose columns can remove the usually more highly anodic IgM, and these eluates can also be concentrated and rerun by IEP. Since immunofixation provides better resolution of the monoclonal component than does IEP, we have found that even cases with relatively small monoclonal IgM gammapathies are easily diagnosed by immunofixation (Figures 5–19 and 5–20).

The easiest and most straightforward approach to this problem was proposed by Penn [66] in a recent ASCP Teleconference. By quantifying the amount of immunoglobulin containing kappa chain and that containing lambda chain (technique follows), one can determine the kappa/lambda ratio of all immunoglobulins in the serum. In most cases where an IgM monoclonal protein exists, the combination of an abnormal kappa/lambda ratio together with the markedly elevated IgM and the obvious spike on HRE should be sufficient to make the diagnosis. For instance, in the case shown in Figures 5–21 and 5–22, there is an obvious area of restricted mobility on the HRE strip and a fourfold elevation of IgM. In addition, there is a markedly elevated kappa/lambda ratio. The combination of the HRE pattern with these immunochemical findings makes further serum studies unnecessary. The accompanying immunofixation (Figure 5–21) illustrates well the monoclonal protein for this volume, but was not needed for diagnosis. In addition to providing straightforward information, these diagnostic procedures can be completed during one day. All cases with such obvious monoclonal gammapathies and markedly abnormal kappa/lambda ratios are completed without immunofixation of serum. If there is any question about the diagnosis, immunofixation must be performed. With the combined use of immunoglobulin quantification and immunofixation (when needed), we rarely resort to special treatment or purification to make a diagnosis.

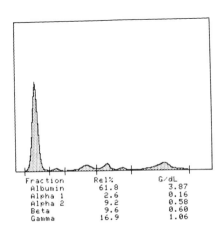

Fraction	Rel%	G/dL
Albumin	61.8	3.87
Alpha 1	2.6	0.16
Alpha 2	9.2	0.58
Beta	9.6	0.60
Gamma	16.9	1.06

Figure 5–19. Densitometric scan shows subtle restriction in the midgamma region.

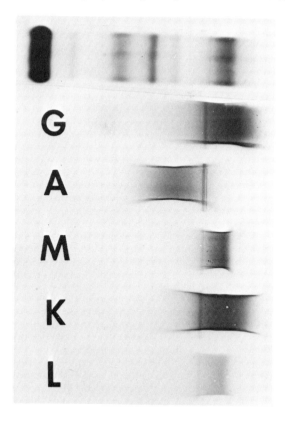

Figure 5-20.   Immunofixation of the serum shown in Figure 5-19 indicates that the restriction is due to an IgM lambda monoclonal protein. (Symbols as in Figure 5-5.)

MONOCLONAL GAMMOPATHIES IN PATIENTS WITH B-LYMPHOCYTE NEOPLASMS

It is clear that plasma cells develop from B lymphocytes (Figure 5-1). Furthermore, patients with myeloma are known to have B cells with surface immunoglobulin and even pre-B cells with cytoplasmic mu of the same idiotype (roughly equivalent with reactivity), implying that although the neoplasm is expressing itself mainly as monoclonal plasma cells, there is really a basic abnormality of that clone throughout the B-cell lineage [16,67]. Finally, B-cell neoplasms such as chronic lymphocytic leukemia have been reported to transform to a predominantly plasma cell neoplasm while producing the same heavy and light chain types, and some cases of myeloma may evolve into an aggressive lymphoproliferative phase characterized by rapidly enlarging soft-tissue masses [68,69].

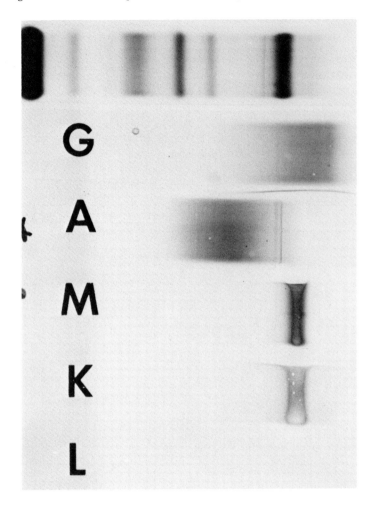

Figure 5-21.   HRE and immunofixation show an obvious IgM kappa monoclonal protein. (Symbols as in Figure 5-5.)

A close relationship between plasma cell neoplasms and B-lymphocyte neoplasms is thus well established. With the application of sensitive techniques such as HRE and immunofixation, it has become clear that most patients with B-cell neoplasms have a monoclonal protein in their serum and/or urine that corresponds to the molecules expressed on their cell surfaces [70]. This should not surprise us; in 1909, Decastello [71] detected Bence Jones protein in the urine from a patient with chronic lymphocytic leukemia. Recent studies with *in vitro* culture proved that B lymphocytes from patients with chronic lymphocytic leukemia (CLL) can be induced, by Epstein-Barr virus or mitogens such as phorbol ester, to differentiate into immunoglobulin-secreting cells [72].

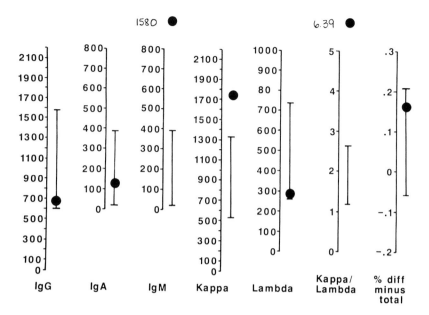

Figure 5–22. The standard chart (after Penn) depicts the values of IgG, IgA, IgM, kappa- and lambda-containing immunoglobulins, and kappa/lambda ratio. There is an obvious increase in IgM and the kappa/lambda ratio. This together with the HRE pattern shown at the top of Figure 5–21 allows us to make the diagnosis of IgM kappa monoclonal gammopathy without performing the immunofixation on serum.

Other CLL cells have been shown to spontaneously secrete monoclonal light chain or monoclonal whole immunoglobulins [73]. The monoclonal globulins found in the serum of patients with CLL are the same molecules that are present on the surface of the neoplastic B lymphocytes [74,75]. Clearly, B-cell CLL and myeloma represent cells from the same lineage at various stages of maturation. The stage of a given B-cell neoplasm is not irreversibly fixed, and may change during the course of an illness.

Other B-cell lymphoproliferative processes have also been reported to show monoclonal proteins in serum or BJP in urine. Nodular lymphoma, Burkitt's lymphoma, and even angioimmunoblastic lymphadenopathy evolving into an immunoblastic lymphoma have had monoclonal proteins demonstrated by a combination of HRE and immunofixation techniques [76–79]. It should be noted, however, that angioimmunoblastic lymphadenopathy is usually characterized by a polyclonal increase in gamma globulins [80]. In some cases, the specific reactivity of the monoclonal protein has produced symptoms useful in characterizing the specific reactivity. For example, patients with some lymphoproliferative disorders can produce a monoclonal antibody against erythrocyte antigens with cold agglutinin activity. Most often this is an IgMK directed against I antigen; although IgML also occurs with this specificity. These proteins frequently occur as cryoglobulins and may have other non-I specificity [81,82]. As discussed later, patients without B-cell lymphoproliferative processes have also had specific reactivity of the monoclonal protein determined. In patients with autoimmune disease, monoclonal antibodies to IgG (monoclonal rheumatoid factor) and to nuclear antigens may be seen.

Monoclonal Gammopathy Associated with Amyloidosis

Amyloidosis is another major clinical condition associated with monoclonal gammopathies. About 4% of patients with plasma cell dyscrasias will have amyloid deposition. Two major biochemical types of amyloid have been recognized in recent years: (1) amyloid consisting of part of an immunoglobulin light chain (AL), and (2) amyloid composed of protein A (AA) [83,84]. AA is probably a subunit or breakdown product of the much larger normal serum molecule, serum amyloid A-related protein (SAA). Patients with secondary amyloidosis associated with chronic infections or rheumatoid arthritis have AA deposition [85].

AL and AA both deposit in tissues causing dysfunction of the specific organs involved. Tissues with extensive involvement by either AA or AL will stain dark blue with iodine (like starch—hence the name *amyloid,* meaning starchlike) and they will stain with Congo red giving a characteristic blue-green birefringence with polarized light. It is now clear that these tinctorial qualities relate to the beta pleated-sheet structure of both AL and AA [86].

In amyloidosis associated with monoclonal gammopathies, the monoclonal component may be subtle or may be a prominent serum and/or urine protein. It is not clear why some light chains are more likely to result in amyloid deposition than others. While the amyloid often is composed of the variable portion of the light chain, this is not always the case; immunohistochemical studies have also demonstrated delta heavy chain in the tissues [25]. The propensity to deposit as amyloid may represent an abnormal synthesis or a degradation product [83].

Tissue deposition of AL preferentially involves the tongue, heart, gastrointestinal tract, blood vessels, tendons, skin, and peripheral nerves. The clinical picture in these patients parallels the sites of involvement, with macroglossia, congestive heart failure, carpal tunnel syndrome, purpura, renal failure, and peripheral neuropathy as prominent features. Further, the optimal sites (which should be judged on the symptoms for the individual case) for biopsies of suspected cases reflect distribution and availability of the site. These patients usually do not have bone pain or osteolytic lesions [87]. Kyle and Greipp [88] recorded 229 patients with AL of whom 47 (20.5%) had multiple myeloma; they found that the presence of myeloma did not contribute to prediction of survival at 1 year. Using the older five-band electrophoretic technique, Kyle and Greipp [88] found a discrete band in only 40% of their patients while demonstrating monoclonal protein in 68% of the sera by IEP; about 70% had Bence Jones proteinuria by IEP. It is certain that the increased resolution of the electrophoretic techniques reviewed in this volume together with immunofixation will increase these percentages.

Monoclonal Gammopathies Not Associated with B-Lymphoproliferative Disorders

Monoclonal gammopathies have been found occasionally in patients with autoimmune diseases. In some cases such as monoclonal antirheumatoid factor and antinuclear antibody, the specificity of the autoantibody is known. In other cases, the relationship of the monoclonal antibody to the autoimmune disease is not known. However, removal of the monoclonal antibody by plasmapheresis has been reported to result in clinical improvement in patients with monoclonal gammopathies associated with polymyositis (where monoclonal antibodies have been detected in the sarcolemmal basement membrane) [89]. We hasten to point out that many other antibodies and nonimmunoglobulin molecules with significant biologic activity are also removed by this process. Which (if any) is responsible for the clinical improvement remains to be determined.

In addition to autoantibodies, monoclonal proteins have reactivity to other common antigens. A wide variety of reactivities of monoclonal proteins that have been determined include bacterial proteins, cardiolipin, polysaccharides, viral antigens, and other major serum proteins including isoenzymes, albumin, and alpha-1 antitrypsin [90–92] (Figure 5–11).

Association of monoclonal gammopathies with peripheral neuropathy has recently been emphasized. While the relationship between the monoclonal gammopathy and the peripheral neuropathy is unclear in most cases, autoreactivity with myelin has been shown [93–95] in some. One specific protein reactivity that has been characterized, called myelin-associated glycoprotein (MAG), has a molecular weight of about 100,000 [96]. Both motor and sensory impairments have been associated with monoclonal gammopathies, and some cases show dramatic improvement following plasmapheresis. Some of these monoclonal proteins may be quite small, requiring immunofixation for adequate demonstration.

Occasional monoclonal gammopathies have been reported in patients with epithelial malignancies. Pick et al. [1] found the most prevalent epithelial tumors associated with monoclonal gammopathies to be gastrointestinal and urinary tract epithelial neoplasms. Of course, the monoclonal proteins were being produced by plasma cells and not the epithelial tumors. The most prevalent isotype associated with epithelial neoplasms was IgM, which occurred in 17 of 52 patients with Waldenstrom's macroglobulinemia in Pick's series [1]. It is unclear whether there is any specific relationship between the two neoplasms in a single individual.

Monoclonal Gammopathy
of Undetermined Significance

While many cases of monoclonal gammopathies fall into one of the categories just discussed, we are profoundly ignorant about the significance of most. A monoclonal gammopathy is demonstrable in the serum of about 1% of individuals over the age of 25 [97,98], but it is unusual for such monoclonal gammopathies to develop into multiple myeloma (incidence, 4 of 100,000) [99].

The incidence of monoclonal gammopathies increases with advancing age, paralleling an increase in polyclonal immunoglobulins [100,101]. IgG- and IgA-containing cells increase considerably in the bone marrow during aging. Most of these cells are probably producing antibodies against exogenous antigens, since their numbers are significantly fewer in germ-free animals [102].

Although the cause of this increased incidence of monoclonal gammopathies with age is unknown, it is clear that immunoregulatory capability also declines with age [103]. Regulatory deficiencies of T-suppressor activity could allow emergence of clonal proliferations, resulting in monoclonal gammopathies [104]. It is also unclear how or even if a benign monoclonal gammopathy evolves into a malignant process; hence the term monoclonal gammopathy of undetermined significance (MGUS). Since the average ages of individuals with myeloma and MGUS are similar (MGUS, 62 years; myeloma, 61 years), epidemiologists have argued that in most cases an evolution into myeloma is unlikely. Nonetheless, as the natural history of any one such lesion is unclear, the clinician must follow such patients closely to determine if the monoclonal protein and/or the clinical course changes. As discussed in following sections, anecdotal cases followed for as long as more than two decades have evolved into multiple myeloma.

There is also laboratory data that implies MGUS is a different disease from myeloma. In patients with MGUS, there are normal numbers of peripheral blood B lymphocytes, whereas in myeloma the numbers of circulating B lymphocytes are decreased [55,105]. Also, the generation time for bone marrow cells in myeloma is considerably faster than that for patients with benign monoclonal gammopathies [106]. A close look at the specificity of the antibody on the B-lymphocyte surface (idiotype) discloses that myeloma patients have B lymphocytes demonstrable in the peripheral blood with antibody of the same idiotype as the myeloma protein, which is not true for most MGUS patients [14]. Other surface marker studies have suggested that the T4-"helper"-cell population is decreased in myeloma but not in MGUS [107].

To diagnose myeloma, one must document the presence of increased plasma cells, tissue involvement, and monoclonality [108]. Kyle and Greipp [109] noted that some patients with these features did not undergo progressive deterioration; they did not have anemia, lytic bone lesions, hypercalcemia, or renal failure. Even though the median initial monoclonal protein was 3.1 g/liter, overt symptoms of myeloma did not develop for at least 5 years of follow-up. They termed the disease of these individuals "smoldering multiple myeloma'' and recommended following them closely without therapy. Other investigators have been even more reserved; Kanoh et al. [110] reported a case with 3-4 g/dl of IgGK monoclonal protein and 10% plasma cells in the bone marrow. Although the patient was mildly anemic (hemoglobin 10.2%), he was otherwise well and was followed with no disease progression for more than two decades.

Clearly, it is not always possible to categorize patients as having myeloma or MGUS. There are many reported cases in the literature in which a patient with a small monoclonal protein was followed for several years, sometimes longer than two decades, before the condition "evolved" into clear-cut myeloma. We have seen a case in which a solitary plasmacytoma was removed, and 17 years later a monoclonal protein of the same isotype was detected in the serum. Therefore, although most patients with MGUS will not evolve, it is important to follow these patients every 6-12 months with a serum or urine protein electrophoresis (depending on the location of their gammopathy) to determine if the disease is evolving. When a monoclonal gammopathy is detected for the first time, the patient needs to have a physical examination, laboratory evaluation for hemoglobin, hematocrit, white blood cell count and differential, calcium, bone marrow examination, skeletal X-rays, and examination of tissue lesions for the conditions we discussed.

Cryoglobulins and Other Monoclonals That May Be Missed

Not all cryoglobulins, which are immunoglobulins that aggregate and precipitate or gel variably at temperatures lower than 37°C, are monoclonal proteins. These are classified by the types of molecules involved (Table 5-2). Type I cryoglobulins are the type most often seen in patients with multiple myeloma or Waldenstrom's macroglobulinemia. In these cases, the monoclonal protein is present in large amounts (>500 mg/dl). Type II cryoglobulins are also associated with monoclonal proteins, but are different from those of type I. These cryoglobulins are an unusual combination of a monoclonal IgM with

Table 5-2 Classification of Cryoglobulins

Type	Composition	Clinical Condition
I	Monoclonal protein	Myeloma, Waldenstrom's
II	Monoclonal IgM and polyclonal IgG	Autoimmune diseases, lymphoproliferative disease, infections
III	Polyclonal IgM and polyclonal IgG, occasionally polyclonal IgA	Autoimmune disease, chronic infections

rheumatoid factor activity that reacts with polyclonal IgG. These proteins are present in much lower concentration than those of type I, and are most often found in patients with autoimmune or lymphoproliferative diseases. Type III cryoglobulins, most frequently encountered and unrelated to monoclonal proteins, consist of polyclonal rheumatoid factor that reacts with polyclonal IgG. Typically, the rheumatoid factor is IgM and the cryoglobulin is present in low concentration (< 100 mg/dl) [111].

Cryoglobulins may be missed by electrophoretic analysis, especially if they precipitate at relatively high temperatures. If proper precautions are not taken in handling the specimen, the cryoglobulin will precipitate during the clotting process and will be missed by electrophoresis or when the sample is placed in the cold. To detect cryoglobulins, the specimen should be drawn in a prewarmed syringe. To maintain the temperature during transportation to the laboratory, some place the sample close to the body such as under an armpit, in a pocket, or worse! However, when the patient cannot be readily transported to the laboratory, we recommend using a thermos and sand, which can easily be kept in a 37°C incubator. This gives excellent thermal stability when compared to 37°C water in a styrofoam cup, and has resulted in improved yield of cryoglobulins [112] (Figure 5-23).

Samples are then processed according to the flow chart (Figure 5-24). The clot must be separated at 37°C and the specimen split into two equal fractions. After azide is added to prevent growth of microorganisms, one fraction is kept at 37°C and the other at 4°C. Samples are examined daily for a week. When a precipitate is seen in the 4°C tube and not in the 37°C tube, it is characterized for total protein, immunoglobulin, and monoclonality. Electrophoresis on a patient with a cryoglobulin is likely to result in a precipitate at the origin (Figure 5-25). Finding such a precipitate should prompt one to investigate the patient for cryoglobulin, monoclonal gammopathy, and circulating immune complexes (Figure 5-26).

Monoclonal proteins other than cryoglobulins can create diagnostic dilemmas for the clinical laboratory. Tetrameric light chain disease can be missed because the serum spike is often in the beta region, where it may be confused with other proteins, and because of molecular size the light chains do not appear in the urine as Bence Jones proteins. Fibrinogen in an incompletely clotted specimen may be mistaken for a monoclonal protein (Figure 5-27). This error will be avoided by looking at the kappa/lambda ratio, checking the serum for a clot (if a small one is present, it indicates that some fibrinogen was left), and repeating the sample (always the best choice when one is not certain of the diagnosis). Further, immunofixation will reveal the true nature of the protein.

Small monoclonal proteins and those monoclonal proteins that migrate in the beta and alpha-2 region are the most difficult to detect. Using a five-band serum protein electrophoresis technique, Kyle [17] reported that 50% of patients with alpha heavy chain disease had a normal pattern. No large studies

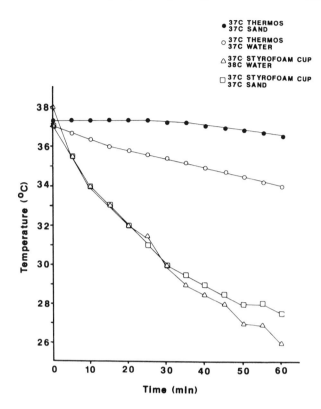

Figure 5–23. Thermal stability of water under the conditions indicated. When water is stored in a thermos containing sand, there is almost no change in temperature up to 1 hour. Thus, we use a thermos with sand, which is stored in a 37°C incubator, to transport samples from patients suspected of having a cryoglobulinemia. Before sampling, the house officers pick up a thermos to use for transporting the patient's sample to the clinical laboratory.

are available for HRE, but the improved resolution should help in the discrimination of smaller gammopathies from transferrin (elevated in iron deficiency), alpha-2 macroglobulin (elevated in the nephrotic syndrome), and large polyclonal increases in gamma such as occur in chronic infections or hepatitis.

Nonsecretory osteosclerotic myelomas are uncommon and require biopsy for diagnosis [113]. In addition, special studies such as column purifications or SDS-polyacrylamide gel electrophoresis may be used to detect small monoclonals or gamma chain disease [114]. The rarity of such cases precludes the clinical laboratory from setting up these costly, specialized studies for this diagnosis. When suspicious cases have inconclusive findings, serum can be sent to a referral center for these more extensive studies.

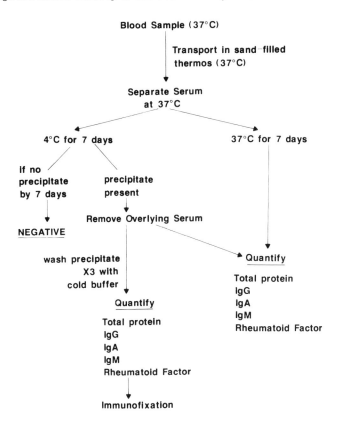

Figure 5–24.   Flow chart used at the University of Michigan for characterizing cryoglobulin samples.

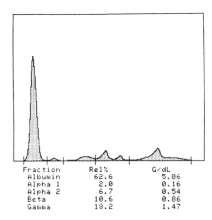

Figure 5–25.   A discrete band is noted at the origin of this densitometric scan. Such bands are usually seen in patients with cryoglobulinemia.

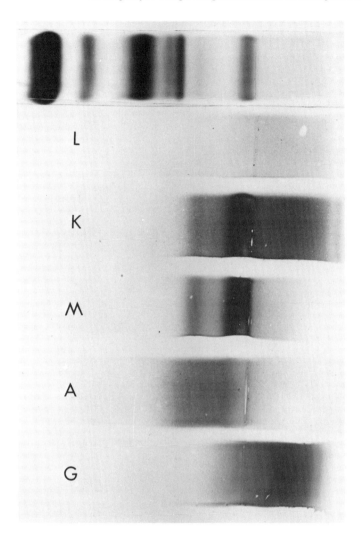

Figure 5-26. Immunofixation of serum from Figure 5-23. This characterizes the cryoglobulin as a monoclonal IgM kappa protein. Note that a faint IgM kappa band is seen anodal to the precipitate at the origin. Not all of the cryoglobulin has precipitated at the origin. (Symbols as in Figure 5-5.)

LABORATORY DIAGNOSIS OF MONOCLONAL GAMMOPATHIES

The major reason for incorporating the techniques of high-resolution electrophoresis (HRE) and immunofixation into the clinical laboratory is to improve the detection of the previously mentioned conditions. Kyle [17] has pointed

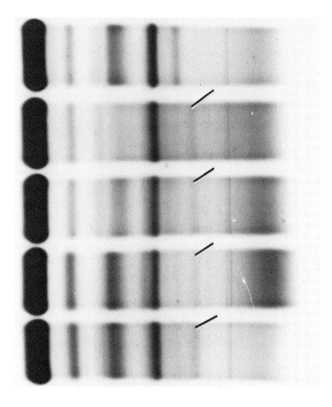

Figure 5-27.   Several samples show a fibrinogen band (*indicated*) because the samples were not allowed to clot completely.

out that resolution is the key for detecting monoclonal proteins, and careful study of the literature corroborates this. For instance, in an extensive study of extramedullary plasmacytomas by Wiltshaw [115] using five-band electrophoresis and IEP, only 1 of 19 patients with this lesion had a *detectable* serum protein gammopathy. On follow-up, however, at least 6 patients developed detectable lesions with these older methods, indicating that the problem with early detection was a lack of sensitivity. As the plasma cell mass increased with time, the amount of secretion became detectable by these less sensitive techniques.

Kappa/Lambda Quantification and the Diagnosis of Monoclonal Gammopathies

The normal ratio of kappa-containing immunoglobulins to lambda-containing immunoglobulins in the serum is 2:1. By using radial immunodiffusion or nephelometric techniques, one can quickly and inexpensively quantify these immunoglobulins. In our own study of control individuals we found that the normal range for kappa/lambda ratio in the serum is 1.2–2.6 (±2 SD). When patients have a chronic infectious disease with a marked elevation of immunoglobulins, such as occurs in osteomyelitis or chronic active hepatitis, there is a polyclonal expansion of B-cell clones. In these conditions, although the total amounts of kappa and lambda are elevated, the kappa/lambda ratio is in the normal range. In contrast, when a monoclonal gammopathy is present, usually there is a marked alteration in the kappa/lambda ratio [116,117]. This results from the combined effect of the marked increase in the monoclonal protein of the single light chain type and the suppression of normal polyclonal immunoglobulin-secreting clones that occurs in myeloma.

Recently, Gerald Penn [116] suggested that by putting together the information gathered by HRE, kappa/lambda quantification, and the clinical picture one could make the correct diagnosis of monoclonal gammopathy within 1 day in most cases. For example, in the case shown in Figures 5–28 and 5–29, there is a marked increase in IgG and kappa, a markedly abnormal kappa/lambda ratio, and a HRE strip that shows a large restricted band in the midgamma region. The diagnosis is an IgG kappa monoclonal gammopathy. Immunofixation or IEP would be an expensive, redundant exercise. As is true in all cases of monoclonal gammopathy identified in the serum, urine IEP for Bence Jones proteins should be performed.

One can even suggest the presence of light chain disease by this technique. The total of IgG, IgA, and IgM concentrations in the serum accounts for more than 99% of the total of kappa- and lambda-containing immunoglobulins under normal circumstances. Therefore, the difference of these two numbers should be close to zero. When the difference of these divided by the total (IgG + IgA + IgM) differs markedly from an established normal range, either light chain disease is present (a large negative number) or there is a difficulty in the technique (perhaps due to aggregation of immunoglobulins). The formula for this calculation is:

$$\frac{(\text{IgG} + \text{IgA} + \text{IgM}) - (\text{kappa} + \text{lambda})}{(\text{IgG} + \text{IgA} + \text{IgM})}$$

We only use this as a rough guide since this formula does not always pick up light chain disease and an abnormal result is occasionally seen in patients without monoclonal gammopathesis.

It is important to use a common sense approach to the evaluation of a monoclonal gammopathy. When first using this technique, we suggest that you perform the redundant immunofixation in obvious cases. One will quickly become used to making this diagnosis with only the HRE and immunoglobulin quantification (including kappa/lambda data). We still perform immunofix-

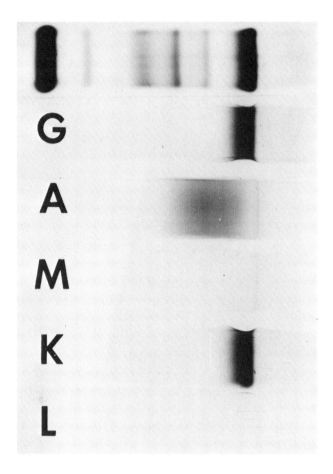

Figure 5-28.   HRE reveals an obvious midgamma band that immunofixation has characterized as an IgG kappa monoclonal gammopathy. (Symbols as in Figure 5-5.)

ation in any case where the diagnosis is not completely obvious; the normal kappa/lambda range of 1.2–2.6 is not used as an absolute cutoff. We have seen cases in which the kappa/lambda was abnormal but no obvious monoclonal band was present. Immunofixation disclosed no monoclonal band in most of these cases. However, in one case (Figure 5-30) the abnormal ratio provided key information. Immunofixation is more sensitive than HRE, and a mildly distorted kappa/lambda ratio could be significant. We have also seen cases of small monoclonal gammopathies in which HRE showed small but obvious discrete bands, but a normal kappa/lambda ratio was present; immunofixation revealed the true monoclonal nature of the lesion (Figures 5-31 and 5-32).

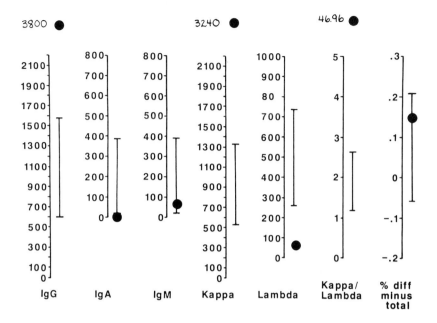

Figure 5–29.   This chart shows the immunoglobulin quantifications for the case seen in Figure 5–28. The IgG kappa monoclonal gammopathy is obvious.

Strategies for Diagnosis of Monoclonal Gammopathies

We suggest the following systematic approach for the correct diagnosis of monoclonal gammopathy with a minimum of time and laboratory work. This approach makes good clinical, laboratory, and economic sense, but we caution the interpreter to be very conservative in his/her approach to these lesions; whenever uncertain about the diagnosis, use more extensive tests, repeat the evaluation on a second sample, or send the serum to a reference laboratory. Most cases will not require these more extensive procedures. Indeed, the best single help in a difficult case is calling on the clinician to correlate your findings with the clinical picture.

The overall strategy is outlined in Table 5–3. If the clinician asks for evaluation for myeloma or any other monoclonal gammopathy (including amyloid, or on samples from patients with symptoms of neuropathy, back pain, etc.), we perform our routine HRE screening test and quantification of IgG, IgA, IgM, kappa, and lambda. If both the HRE and the immunoglobulin quantifications (including the kappa/lambda ratio) are normal, we report that the serum and immunoglobulins are normal. With a pertinent clinical history, we also recommend study of the urine for BJP if light chain disease is part of the differential diagnosis.

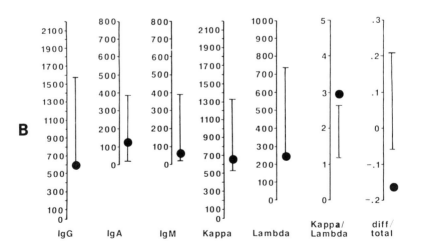

Figure 5-30.   A. Small area of restricted mobility is, at best, faintly seen in the mid-gamma region of the HRE strip. However, immunofixation revealed a definite kappa monoclonal band (*indicated*). B. Chart shows the immunoglobulin quantifications from this patient. Note that the kappa/lambda ratio was abnormal.

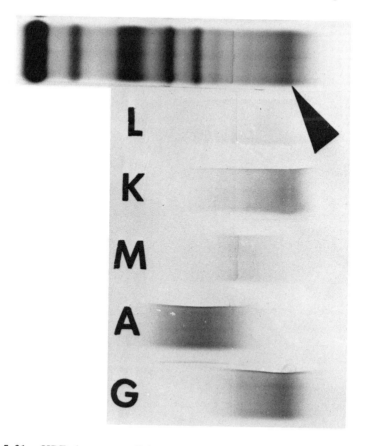

Figure 5–31. HRE shows a small but definite midgamma restriction. The immuno-fixation indicates that this is an IgG kappa monoclonal gammopathy.

Table 5–3   Strategy for Evaluation of Serum for Monoclonal Gammopathies

HRE	Kappa/Lambda Ratio[a]	Further Test	Diagnosis	Time (days)
Normal	Normal	None	Normal	1
Polyclonal	Normal	None	Polyclonal	1
M component	Abnormal	None	Specific IgX	1
M component	Normal	Immunofixation	Specific IgX	2

[a]Normal or borderline kappa/lambda ratio requires immunofixation when a restriction is seen.

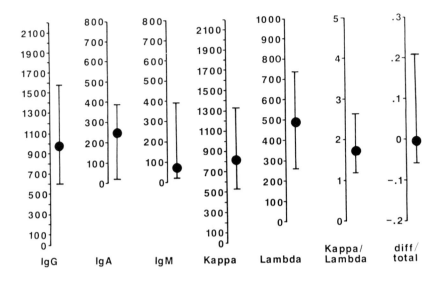

Figure 5-32. Chart shows the immunoglobulin quantifications from the case shown in Figure 5-31. Note that the kappa/lambda ratio is normal. When small monoclonal gammopathies are present together with normal or elevated polyclonal immunoglobulins, the kappa/lambda ratio will be unreliable for making the final diagnosis.

The serum HRE is key to this approach. A low gamma globulin region is often ignored, and some erroneously believe this is a normal finding in older individuals. False! Older individuals usually have normal immunoglobulin concentrations. Total B-cell number and immunoglobulin content are the same in older individuals as in young [118]. This erroneous impression is partly because some specific antibody levels do differ. Due to a decreased suppressor-T-cell function and altered helper function, more autoantibodies are seen, whereas the response elicited to foreign antigens is often weak [119,120]. Hypogammaglobulinemia (which we usually diagnose by densitometric scan of the gamma region) (see Chapter 2) is an important tip-off that the patient may have light chain disease or one of the B-cell neoplasms listed above. When hypogammaglobulinemia is seen, immunofixation should be performed on the serum and IEP on the urine to detect the small monoclonals that are seen with B-cell neoplasms or the BJP found in light chain disease. Other abnormalities in the serum must be carefully examined. A low albumin is suspicious; a restriction in any portion of the protein electrophoresis is not normal. However, when patients have an obvious polyclonal increase in gamma without restriction and a normal kappa/lambda ratio, we sign out the sample as a polyclonal increase in the specific globulins elevated. If there is an obvious restriction in the HRE pattern and an obvious abnormality in the kappa/lambda ratio, we interpret the monoclonal gammopathy and request a urine to determine if Bence Jones proteinuria accompanies the monoclonal protein.

When the physician has sent a serum sample as a screen, with no clinical evidence for monoclonal gammopathy (by history), a routine HRE is performed. Any abnormal band from the alpha-1 through the gamma region is regarded with suspicion. Most can be interpreted by understanding the pattern diagnoses outlined in Chapter 3. A nephrotic patient can have a markedly elevated alpha-2 macroglobulin, and an iron-deficient patient will have an elevated transferrin band. Any unexplained band should cause the interpreter to inform the clinician about the abnormal pattern and perform immunoglobulin quantification. As stated earlier, a low gamma region should be considered an important finding as it may indicate an immune deficiency, a lymphoplasmacytic neoplasm, or the effect of chemotherapy. It is not normal, and one must inform the clinician and recommend a urine to rule out BJP.

When one is consulted about the results of general chemistry laboratory screening for an individual patient, a low albumin, elevated calcium, elevated total protein, or decreased albumin/globulin ratio are sufficient abnormalities to recommend HRE of serum with quantification of immunoglobulins (including kappa/lambda). Information about such chemical abnormalities should raise your level of suspicion when viewing an HRE pattern. Similarly, routine hematologic screening tests that demonstrate plasma cells on the differential, Rouleaux formation on the blood smear, or a bone marrow with >10% plasma cells should be considered suspicious. These relevant laboratory findings should result in HRE and quantifications of immunoglobulin with kappa/lambda ratio.

To conserve time and important laboratory resources, it is important to maintain a file on all monoclonal proteins detected. When a sample is received with a request to evaluate for monoclonal protein, the old file is quickly checked for any previous findings in the same patient [118]. An HRE is performed on serum, and the monoclonal band (if in the gamma region) is quantified by densitometry [119]. If there is no change in pattern, there is no reason to perform kappa/lambda quantification or immunofixation. You have helped the clinicians follow the patient by determining the change (if any) of the monoclonal protein quantity, and you have provided this information quickly. As there was no need to perform the redundant immunofixation assay, laboratory reagent and technologist time has not been wasted performing kappa/lambda ratios already known to be abnormal. If the patient has a beta- or alpha-migrating monoclonal lesion, HRE and quantification of the specific heavy chain are needed to follow the patient. Because of the other proteins in these regions (alpha-2 macroglobulin, haptoglobin, transferrin, and C3), densitometric scanning is impracticable to quantify any change in monoclonal protein.

If the patient has light chain disease, 24-hour urine should be collected, total protein determined, and densitometry used to establish the percentage of

BJP. Obviously, tetrameric light chain disease must be followed by serum samples as the molecules are too large to pass into the urine [120]. Any change in the electrophoretic migration or the development of other suspicious bands should trigger a reinvestigation complete with immunofixation to determine if the patient is developing a double gammopathy or if the course of the condition has altered.

When the clinician sends a urine to be evaluated for BJP, we perform HRE on 100-fold concentrated urine. When the urine has considerable protein, it will not readily concentrate to this level. This is of no significance as the goal is the qualitative detection of monoclonal protein. Urine IEP is performed simultaneously. We do not perform immunofixation routinely on urines at the present time; we have found this difficult to set up at optimal concentration for precipitation since the current methods to quantify kappa and lambda in the urine are clumsy. As discussed in Chapter 4, IEP allows for automatic adjustment of the protein concentrations toward equivalence with the reagent antisera as the molecules diffuse through the agarose. With immunofixation, one may be off in concentration as much as 1000-fold in urine; therefore, extreme antibody excess and antigen excess can be problematic. Further, we have often found restrictions that are more likely caused by deteriorations of the molecules in the urine that are seen by immunofixation. This "noise" level makes interpretation difficult. Therefore, until better kappa/lambda quantifications are available for urine, we recommend using IEP to qualitatively detect BJP.

We have found this strategy provides efficient processing of specimens, which benefits the patient, the clinician, and the laboratory. It helps prevent problems of inappropriate ordering and overutilization of the laboratory. Several years ago, we were struck with the large number of normal IEPs that were being performed; many were being requested on children and young adults. On questioning the physicians ordering such tests (usually house officers and fellows, although some senior staff were involved), we found that they were interested in a serum protein electrophoresis screen rather than an evaluation for monoclonal protein. This is a problem in education that is not easily solved. Despite sending many notices about the difference in the procedures, speaking at rounds, and attending many of the clinical conferences, we were unable to significantly reduce the number of such inappropriate tests. The prolonged testing was needlessly expensive to the patient then (and to the institution now), wasted time (a very expensive commodity under newer strategies of payment), and prevented the laboratory from developing other useful tests.

With the incorporation of our strategy, clinicians in our institution have been appreciative of the more rapid turnaround time and, in general, like being involved in the evaluation of problem specimens. An occasional clinician has objected to our finding a small monoclonal protein or a hypogammaglobulinemia without apparent cause. We are not able to determine the meaning of each abnormality detected by these sensitive methods, but we do know (as has been discussed) the important conditions that need to be ruled in or out. When we have a very small monoclonal about which we are uncertain after talking to the clinician and studying the urine, we recommend repeating the evaluation in 6–12 months. If it represents an early malignant monoclonal process, it will still be there or may have progressed to the point where it will be readily detectable. If it was merely an oligoclonal expansion due to some infection or other process, it will likely have resolved by this time.

These approaches are really nothing more than good common sense laboratory medicine to prevent over- and underutilization of laboratory tests. By using these approaches, one will find that the time spent by the laboratory doing needless procedures (such as immunofixation of a 13-year-old girl with an infection) will decrease considerably, and the turnaround time on important specimens will decrease by days in some cases. A cooperative relationship between the laboratory and clinician is one of the critical points to success in such cases. Never be afraid to call for more clinical information and to involve the physician in the decision-making process. When uncertain about a result, repeat the procedure, speak to the clinician, perform further studies, and occasionally send the sample off for reference work. With the techniques and strategies outlined, such referrals will be extremely uncommon.

REFERENCES

1. Pick AI, Shoenfeld Y, Frohlichmann R, Weiss H, Bana D, Schreibman S. Plasma cell dyscrasia. Analysis of 423 patients. JAMA 1979;241:2275–2278.
2. Bruton OC. Agammaglobulinemia. Pediatrics 1952;9:722–727.
3. Glick B, Chang TS, Jaap RG. The bursa of Fabricius and antibody production. Poult Sci 1956;35:224–232.
4. Johnstone AP. Chronic lymphocytic leukaemia and its relationship to normal B lymphopoiesis. Immunol Today 1982;3:343–348.
5. Caligaris-Cappio F, Janossy G. Surface markers in chronic lymphoid leukemia of B cell type. Semin Hematol 1985;22:1–12.
6. Korsmeyer SJ, Greene WC, Cossman J, Hsu SM, Jensen JP, Neckers LM, Marshall SL, Bakhshi A, Depper JM, Leonard WJ, Jaffee ES, Waldmann TA. Rearrangement and expression of immunoglobulin gene and expression of Tac antigen in hairy cell leukemia. Proc Natl Acad Sci USA 1983;80:4511–4526.
7. Hayakawa K, Hardy RR, Parks DR, Herzenberg LA. The "Ly-1 B" cell subpopulation in normal immunodefective and autoimmune mice. J Exp Med 1983;157:202–218.
8. Hayward AR. Development of lymphocyte responses and interactions in human fetuses and newborn. Immunol Rev 1981;57:39–60.
9. Hofman FM, Danilovs J, Husmann L, Taylor CR. Ontogeny of B-cell markers in the human fetal liver. J Immunol 1984;133:1197–1201.
10. Lovett EJ, Schnitzer B, Keren DF, Flint A. Application of flow cytometry to diagnostic pathology. Lab Invest 1984;50:115–140.
11. Reinherz EL, Cooper MD, Schlossman SF, Rosen FS. Abnormalities of T-cell maturation and regulation in human beings with immunodeficiency disorders. J Clin Invest 1981;68:699–705.

12. Foon KA, Schroff RW, Gale RP. Surface markers on leukemia and lymphoma cells: recent advances. Blood 1982;60:1–18.
13. Katagiri S, Yonezawa T, Tamaki T, Kanayama Y, Kuyama J, Ohnishi M, Tsubakio T, Kurata Y, Tarui S. Surface expression of human myeloma cells: an analysis using a panel of monoclonal antibodies. Acta Haematol (Basel) 1984;72:372–378.
14. Bast EJEG, Van Camp B, Reynaert P, Wiriga G, Ballieux RE. Idiotypic blood lymphocytes in monoclonal gammopathies. Clin Exp Immunol 1982;47:677–682.
15. Van Acker A, Conte PF, Hulin N, Rubain J. Idiotypic studies on myeloma B cells. Eur J Cancer 1979;15:627–635.
16. Kubagawa H, Vogler L, Captra JD, Conrad ME, Lawton A, Cooper MD. Studies on the clonal origin of multiple myeloma. J Exp Med 1979;150:792–807.
17. Kyle RA. Multiple myeloma review of 869 cases. Mayo Clin Proc 1975;50:29–40.
18. Schur PH, Kyle RA, Bloch KJ, Hammock WJ, Rivers SL, Sargent A, Ritchie RF, McIntyre OG, Moloney WC, Wolfson AB. IgG subclasses: relationship to clinical aspects of multiple myeloma and frequency distribution among M-components. Scand J Haematol 1974;12:60–68.
19. Hammarstrom L, Mellstedt H, Persson MAA, Smith CIE, Ahre A. IgA subclass distribution in paraproteinemias: suggestion of an IgG-IgA subclass switch pattern. Acta Pathol Microbiol Immunol Scand [C] 1984;92:207–211.
20. Bachman R. The diagnostic significance of the serum concentration of pathological proteins (M-components). Acta Med Scand 1965;178:801–808.
21. Zarrabi MH, Stark RS, Kane P, Dannaher CL, Chandor S. IgM myeloma, a distinct entity in the spectrum of B-cell neoplasia. Am J Clin Pathol 1981;75:1–10.
22. Jancelewicz Z, Takatsuki K, Sugai S, Prozanski W. IgD multiple myeloma review of 133 cases. Arch Intern Med 1975;135:87–93.
23. Vladutiu AO, Nett D. Is quantitation of serum IgD clinically useful? Clin Chem 1982;28:1409–1410.
24. Jennette JC, Wilkman AS, Benson JD. IgD myeloma with intracytoplasmic crystalline inclusions. Am J Clin Pathol 1981;75:231–235.
25. Schaldenbrand JD, Keren DF. IgD amyloid in an IgD lambda monoclonal conjunctival amyloidoma—a case report. Arch Pathol Lab Med 1983;107:626–628.
26. Endo T, Okumura H, Kikuchi K, Munakata J, Otake M, Nomura T, Asakawa H. Immunoglobulin E (IgE) multiple myeloma: a case report and review of the literature. Am J Med 1981;70:1127–1132.
27. Proacter SJ, Chaula SL, Bard AG, Stephenson J. Hyperviscosity syndrome in IgE myeloma. Br Med J 1984;289:1112.
28. Pick AI, Schoenfeld Y, Schreibman S. Asymptomatic monoclonal gammopathies: a study of 100 patients. Ann Clin Lab Sci 1977;7:335–343.
29. Hobbs JR. Paraproteinemia benign or malignant. Br Med J 1967;3:699–704.
30. Solling K, Solling J, Nielsen JS. Polymeric Bence Jones proteins in serum in myeloma patients with renal insufficiency. Acta Med Scand 1984;216:495–502.
31. Clyne DH, Pesce AJ, Thompson RE. Nephrotoxicity of Bence Jones proteins in the rat: importance of protein isoelectric point. Kidney Int 1979;16:345–352.
32. Preud'homme JL, Morel-Maroger L, Brouet JC, Mignon F, Seligmann M. Synthesis of abnormal immunoglobulins in lymphoplasmacytic disorders with visceral light chain deposition. Am J Med 1980;69:703–710.

33. Stone MJ, Frenkel EP. The clinical spectrum of light chain myeloma. Study of 35 patients with special reference to the occurrence of systemic amyloidosis. Am J Med 1975;58:601–619.
34. Shustik C, Bergsagel DE, Pruzanski W. Kappa and lambda light chain disease: survival rates and clinical manifestations. Blood 1976;48:41–51.
35. Horn MF, Knapp MS, Page FT, Walker WHC. Adult Fanconi syndrome and multiple myelomatosis. J Clin Pathol 1969;22:414–416.
36. Hobbs JR. Bence-Jones proteins. Essays Med Biochem 1974;1:105–131.
37. Laurell CB. Complexes formed in vivo between immunoglobulin light chain kappa, prealbumin, and/or alpha-1 antitrypsin in multiple myeloma sera. Immunochemistry 1970;7:461–465.
38. Alanen A, Pira U, Lassila O, Roth J, Franklin RM. Mott cells are plasma cells defective in immunoglobulin secretion. Eur J Immunol 1985;15:235.
39. Preud'homme JL, Hurez D, Danon F, Brouet JC, Seligmann M. Intracytoplasmic and surface-bound immunoglobulins in "nonsecretory" and Bence-Jones myeloma. Clin Exp Immunol 1976;25:428–436.
40. Clark KA, Keren DF. Demonstration of monoclonal lymphoplasmacytic proliferations by immunofluorescence on routine formalin-fixed, paraffin-embedded tissue. Cancer 1982;49:2376–2382.
41. Seligmann M, Rambaud JC. Alpha-chain disease: an immunoproliferative disease of the secretory immune system. Ann NY Acad Sci 1983;409:478–484.
42. Tracey RP, Kyle RA, Leitch JM. Alpha heavy-chain disease presenting as goiter. Am J Clin Pathol 1984;82:336–339.
43. Novis BH, King HS, Gilinsky NH, Mee AS, Young G. Long survival in a patient with alpha-chain disease. Cancer 1984;53:970–973.
44. Al-Saleem TI, Qadiry WA, Issa FS, King J. The immunoselection technic in laboratory diagnosis of alpha heavy-chain disease. Am J Clin Pathol 1979;72:132–133.
45. Guardia J, Rubies-Prat J, Gallart MT, Moragas A, Martinex-Vazquez JM, Bacardi R, Vilasega J. The evolution of alpha heavy chain disease. Am J Med 1976;60:596–602.
46. Franklin EC, Lowenstein J, Bigelow B, Meltzer M. Heavy chain disease. A new disorder of serum gamma-globulins. Report of the first case. Am J Med 1964;37:332–350.
47. Bloch KJ, Lee L, Mills JA, Haber E. Gamma heavy chain disease: an expanding clinical and laboratory spectrum. Am J Med 1973;55:61–70.
48. Lennert K, Mohri N, Stein H, Kaiserling E. The histopathology of malignant lymphoma. Br J Haematol 1975;31:193–203 (Suppl).
49. Ballard HS, Hamilton LM, Marcus AJ, Illes CH. A new variant of heavy-chain disease (mu-chain disease). N Engl J Med 1970;282:1060–1062.
50. Robinson RA, Katzmann JA. The clinical aspects of biclonal gammopathies. Am J Med 1981;71:999–1009.
51. Ritchie RF, Case DC. IgD multiple myeloma: always a near miss. Am Soc Clin Pathol, ASCP Check Sample No. IP 82-8;1982.
52. Bhagavan NV, Scottolini AG. Biclonal IgA and IgM gammopathy in lymphocytic lymphoma. Clin Chem 1984;30:1710–1712.
53. Flanagan JG, Rabbitts T. Arrangement of immunoglobulin heavy chain constant region genes implies evolutionary duplication of a segment containing gamma, epsilon and alpha genes. Nature (London) 1982;300:709–713.

54. Nagai K, Takatsuki K, Uchino H. Clinical significance of immunoglobulin secreting cells in the peripheral blood in patients with multiple myeloma. Scand J Immunol 1983;14:99-105.

55. Pilarski LM, Mant MJ, Reuther BA, Belch A. Severe deficiency of B lymphocytes in peripheral blood from multiple myeloma patients. J Clin Invest 1984;74:1301-1306.

56. Broder S, Humphrey R, Duron M, Blackman M, Meade B, Goldman C, Strober W, Waldman T. Impaired synthesis of polyclonal (non-paraprotein) immunoglobulin by circulating lymphocytes from patients with multiple myeloma. N Engl J Med 1975;293:887-892.

57. Bergmann L, Mitrou PS, Weber KC, Keiker W. Imbalances of T-cell subsets in monoclonal gammopathies. Cancer Immunol Immunother 1984;17:112-116.

58. Levinson AI, Hoxie JA, Matthews DM, Schreiber AD, Negendank WG. Analysis of the relationship between T cell subsets and in vitro B cell responses in multiple myeloma. J Clin Lab Immunol 1985;16:23-26.

59. Tamaki T, Katagiri S, Kanayama Y, Konishi I, Yonezawa T, Tarui S, Kitani T. Helper T-cell lymphoma with marked plasmacytosis and polyclonal hypergammaglobulinemia. A case report. Cancer 1984;53:1590-1595.

60. Chen Y, Bhoopalam N, Yakulis V, Heller P. Changes in lymphocyte surface immunoglobulins in myeloma and the effect of an RNA-containing plasma factor. Ann Intern Med 1975;83:625-631.

61. Chen Y, Hwang LT, Heller P. Immunosuppression in plasmacytoma: induction of suppressor cells. Clin Exp Immunol 1982;47:191-196.

62. Fudenberg HH, Virella G. Multiple myeloma and Waldenstrom's macroglobulinemia: unusual presentations. Semin Hematol 1980;17:63-79.

63. Tichy MM, Blaha M, Siroky O, Vanasek J, Jebavy L, Hencir Z. A case of "acute" Waldenstrom macroglobulinemia. Haematologica 1984;17:125-131.

64. Leonhard SA, Muhleman AF, Hurtibise PE, Martelo OJ. Emergence of immunoblastic sarcoma in Waldenstrom's macroglobulinemia. Cancer 1980;45:3102-3107.

65. Orr KB. Use of 2-mercaptoethanol to facilitate detection and classification of IgM abnormalities by IEP. J Immunol Methods 1979;30:339-349.

66. Penn G. ASCP Teleconference, 1984.

67. Boccadoro M, Van Acker A, Pileri A, Urbain J. Idiotypic lymphocytes in human monoclonal gammopathies. Adv Immunol (Inst Pasteur) 1981;132C:9-19.

68. Pines A, Ben-Bassat I, Selzer G, Ramot B. Transformation of chronic lymphocytic leukemia to plasmacytoma. Cancer 1984;54:1904-1907.

69. Suchman AL, Coleman M, Mornadian JA, Wolf DJ, Saletan S. Aggressive plasma cell myeloma a terminal phase. Arch Intern Med 1981;141:1315-1320.

70. Deegan MJ, Abraham JP, Sawdyk M, Van Slyck EJ. High incidence of monoclonal proteins in the serum and urine of chronic lymphocytic leukemia patients. Blood 1984;6:1207-1211.

71. Decastello AV. Beitrage zur Kenntnis der Bence-Jonesschen Albuminurie. Z Klin Med 1909;67:319-343.

72. Deegan MJ, Maeda K. Differentiation of chronic lymphocytic leukemia cells after in vitro treatment with Epstein-Barr virus or phorbol ester. I. Immunologic and morphologic studies. Am J Hematol 1984;17:335-347.

73. Hannam-Harris AC, Gordon J, Smith SL. Immunoglobulin synthesis by neo-

plastic B lymphocytes: free light chain synthesis as a marker of B cell differentiation. J Immunol 1980;125:2177–2181.

74. Fu SM, Winchester RJ, Feizi T, Walzer PD, Kunkel HG. Idiotypic specificity of surface immunoglobulin and the maturation of leukemic bone-marrow-derived lymphocytes. Proc Natl Acad Sci USA 1974;71:4487–4489.

75. Qian G, Fu SM, Solanki DL, Rai KR. Circulating monoclonal IgM proteins in B cell chronic lymphocytic leukemia: their identification, characterization and relationship to membrane IgM. J Immunol 1984;133:3396–4000.

76. Bauer TW, Mendelsohn G, Humphrey RL, Mann RB. Angioimmunoglastic lymphadenopathy progressing to immunoblastic lymphoma with prominent gastric involvement. Cancer 1982;50:2089–2098.

77. Palutke M, McDonald JM. Monoclonal gammopathies associated with malignant lymphoma. Am J Clin Pathol 1973;60:157–165.

78. Pascali E, Pezzoli A, Melata M, Falconieri G. Nodular lymphoma eventuating into lymphoplasmacytic lymphoma with monoclonal IgM/L cold agglutining and Bence Jones proteinuria. Acta Haematol (Basel) 1980;64:94–102.

79. Braunstein AH, Keren DF. Monoclonal gammopathy (IgM-Kappa) occurring in Burkitt's lymphoma. Arch Pathol Lab Med 1983;107:235–238.

80. Prchal JJ, Crago SS, Mestecky J, Okos AJ, Flint A. Immunoblastic lymphoma: an immunologic study. Cancer 1981;47:2312–2322.

81. Seligmann M, Brouet JC. Antibody activity of human myeloma globulins. Semin Hematol 1973;10:163–177.

82. Roelcke D. Cold agglutination antibodies and antigens. Clin Immunol Immunopathol 1974;2:266–280.

83. Cohen AS. An update of clinical, pathologic and biochemical aspects of amyloidosis. Int J Dermatol 1981;20: 515–530.

84. Levin M, Franklin EC, Frangione B, Pras M. The amino acid sequence of a major nonimmunoglobulin component of some amyloid fibrils. J Clin Invest 1972;51:2773–2776.

85. Skogen B, Thorsteinsson L, Natvig JB. Degradation of protein SAA to an AA-like fragment by enzymes of monocyte origin. Scand J Immunol 1980;11:533–540.

86. Glenner GG. Amyloid deposits and amyloidosis. The beta-fibrilloses. N Engl J Med 1980;302:1283–1292.

87. Pick AI, Frohlichmann R, Lavie G, Duczyminer M, Skvaril F. Clinical and immunochemical studies of 20 patients with amyloidosis and plasma cell dyscrasia. Acta Haematol (Basel) 1981;66:154–167.

88. Kyle RA, Greipp PR. Amyloidosis (AL) clinical and laboratory features in 229 cases. Mayo Clin Proc 1983;58:665–683.

89. Kiprox DD, Miller RG. Polymyositis associated with monoclonal gammopathy. Lancet 1984;ii:1183–1186.

90. Seligmann M, Brouet JC. Antibody activity of human myeloma globulins. Semin Hematol 1973;10:163–177.

91. Potter M. Myeloma proteins (M-components) with antibody-like activity. N Engl J Med 1971;284:831–839.

92. Laurell CB. Complexes formed in vivo between immunoglobulin light chain kappa, prealbumin, and/or alpha 1-antitrypsin in myeloma sera. Immunochemistry 1970;7:461–465.

93. Latov N, Sherman WH, Nemni R, Galassi G, Shyong J, Penn AS, Chess L, Olarte RR, Rowland LP, Osserman EF. Plasma cell dyscrasia and peripheral neuropathy with a monoclonal antibody to peripheral nerve myelin. N Engl J Med 1980;303:618–621.

94. Driedger H, Pruzanski W. Plasma cell neoplasia with peripheral neuropathy. Medicine 1980;59:301–310.

95. Dalakas MC, Engel WK. Polyneuropathy with monoclonal gammopathy: studies of 11 patients. Ann Neurol 1981;10:45–52.

96. Steck AJ, Murray N, Meier C, Page N, Perrusseau G. Demyelinating neuropathy and monoclonal IgM antibody to myelin-associated glycoprotein. Neurology 1983;33:19–23.

97. Fine JM, Lambin P, Lerous P. Frequency of monoclonal gammopathy in 13,400 sera from blood donors. Vox Sang 1976;23:336–340.

98. Axelsson U, Bachmann R, Hallen J. Frequency of pathological proteins (M-components) in 6,995 sera from an adult population. Acta Med Scand 1966;179:235–242.

99. Kyle RA. Monoclonal gammopathy of undetermined significance (MGUS): a review. Clin Haematol 1982;11:123–150.

100. Buckley CE, Dorsey FC. The effect of aging on human serum immunoglobulin concentration. J Immunol 1970;105:964–972.

101. Kishimoto S, Tomino S, Inomata K, Kotegawa S, Saito T, Kuroki M, Mitsuya H, Hisamatsu S. Age-related changes in the subsets and functions of human T lymphocytes. J Immunol 1978;121:1773–1780.

102. Benner R, Hijimans W, Haaijman JJ. The bone marrow: the major source of immunoglobulins, but still a neglected site of antibody formation. Clin Exp Immunol 1981;46:1–8.

103. Makinodan T, Kay MMB. Age influence on the immune system. Adv Immunol 1980;29:287–330.

104. Radl J. Differences among the three major categories of paraproteinemias in aging man and the mouse. A minireview. Mech Ageing Devel 1984;28:167–170.

105. Lindstrom FD, Hardy WR, Eberle BJ, Williams RC. Multiple myeloma and benign monoclonal gammopathy: differentiation by immunofluorescence of lymphocytes. Ann Intern Med 1973;78:837–844.

106. Durie BGM, Salmon SE, Moon TE. Pretreatment of tumor mass, cell kinetics and prognosis in multiple myeloma. Blood 1980;55:364–372.

107. Bergmann L, Mitrou PS, Kelker W, Weber KC. T-cell subsets in malignant lymphomas and monoclonal gammopathies. Scand J Haematol 1985;34:170–176.

108. Committee of the Chronic Leukemia-Myeloma Task Force, National Cancer Institute. Proposed guidelines for protocol studies. II. Plasma cell myeloma. Cancer Chemother Rep 1973;4(part 3):145–158.

109. Kyle RA, Greipp PR. Smoldering multiple myeloma. N Engl J Med 1980;302:1347–1349.

110. Kanoh T, Koya M, Uchino H. Smoldering multiple myeloma associated with anemia. N Engl J Med 1985;312:1192–1193.

111. Keren DF. Assays for circulating immune complexes. In: Homburger HA, Batsakis JB, eds. Clinical laboratory annual: 1985. Norwalk: Appleton-Century/ Crofts, 1985:105–142.

112. Keren DF, DiSante AC, Mervak T, Bordine SL. Problems with transporting

serum to the laboratory for cryoglobulin assay: a solution. Clin Chem 1985;31: 1766–1767.

113. Raman S, Frame B, Saeed SM, Tolia K, Raju U, Kottamasu S. Diffuse nonsecretory osteosclerotic myeloma with extensive phagocytosis. Am J Clin Pathol 1983;80:84–88.

114. Ruiz-Arguelles A, Valls-de-Ruiz M, Ruiz-Arguelles GJ. On excluding monoclonal gammopathy. Am J Clin Pathol 1984;81:409–410.

115. Wiltshaw E. The natural history of extramedullary plasmacytoma and its relation to solitary myeloma of bone and myelomatosis. Medicine 1976;55:217–238.

116. Perry MB, Hayashi H. Kappa and lambda ratios by rate nephelometry to screen and monitor paraproteins. Fed Proc 39;1980:920.

117. Tichy M, Hrncir Z. Diagnostic significance of kappa/lambda and lambda/kappa ratio in paraproteinemias. Supplementum Sborniku vedeckych praci Lekarske fakulty UK v Hradci Kralove 1982;25:3/4:313–318.

118. Rao KMK, Bordine SL, Keren DF. Decision making by pathologists: a strategy for curtailing inappropriate tests. Arch Pathol Lab Med 1982;106:55–56.

119. Keren DF, Di Sante AC, Bordine SL. Densitometric scanning of high-resolution electrophoresis of serum: methodology and clinical application. Am J Clin Pathol 1986;85:348–352.

120. Hom BL. Polymeric (presumed tetrameric) lambda Bence Jones proteinemia without proteinuria in a patient with multiple myeloma. Am J Clin Pathol 1984;82:627–629.

CHAPTER 6

Case Studies for Interpretation

The principles of high-resolution electrophoresis and immunofixation have been reviewed in the preceding chapters, and the specific bands and patterns have been outlined. This chapter allows the reader to interpret some cases from our files. In most of these cases, we only knew the age and sex of the individual at the time of the initial interpretation. Readers should review the electrophoretic information and make their interpretation and, where appropriate, their suggestions for the clinician. Our discussion follows each series of cases. In the first group of cases, the gels were stained with Amido black and scanned by densitometry as described in the text (Figures 6-1 through 6-8). The immunofixation samples (Figures 6-9 through 6-19) were stained with Coomassie blue, which gives a darker staining than the Amido black and is more sensitive (Chapter 2). However, we cannot scan these for densitometric information.

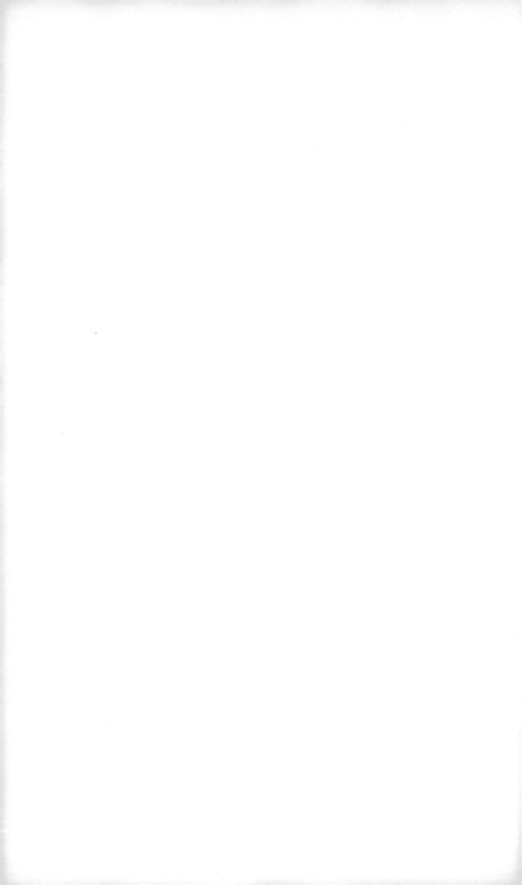

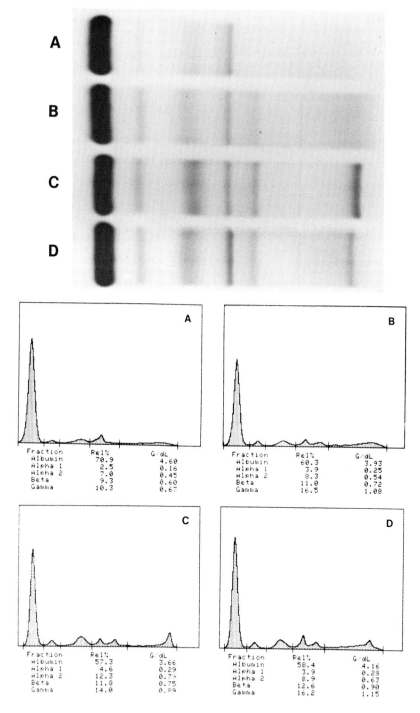

Figure 6–1. Case A: No clinical information. Dade. Case B: 23-year-old man. Case C: 47-year-old man. Case D: 52-year-old woman.

Interpretation for Figure 6-1

Case A. This is a typical lyophilized control sample. The most notable features include the absence of a C3 band due to its activation with the formation of C3c. Also, the gamma globulin region is borderline low by densitometry and looks relatively faint by direct vision.

Case B. This is a normal pattern.

Case C. There is a definite band in the slow gamma region, and the gamma globulin other than the band appears relatively faint. A file, which should be double checked, should be kept on all patients with demonstrated monoclonal gammopathies. If the patient does not have a known monoclonal gammopathy, quantification of IgG, IgA, IgM, kappa, and lambda should be performed. In such cases, the clinician is informed of the gammopathy. The differential diagnosis of such small monoclonals reviewed in Chapter 5 is discussed. In this case, the patient had a peripheral neuropathy. Further studies revealed a monoclonal IgM kappa gammopathy. It is unusual for an IgM to migrate this cathodally, but monoclonal gammopathies associated with peripheral neuropathies are often IgM.

Case D. There is a definite, although small, slow gamma band. Unlike Case C (Figure 6-1C), the remainder of the gamma globulin region was relatively normal. Nonetheless, we called the clinician to inform him of this band and to obtain more clinical information; the sample had been sent as part of a routine screen. Immunofixation revealed a small monoclonal IgG kappa gammopathy, the kappa/lambda ratio was normal, and the subsequent clinical workup was negative. This monoclonal gammopathy of undetermined significance (MGUS) is being followed annually.

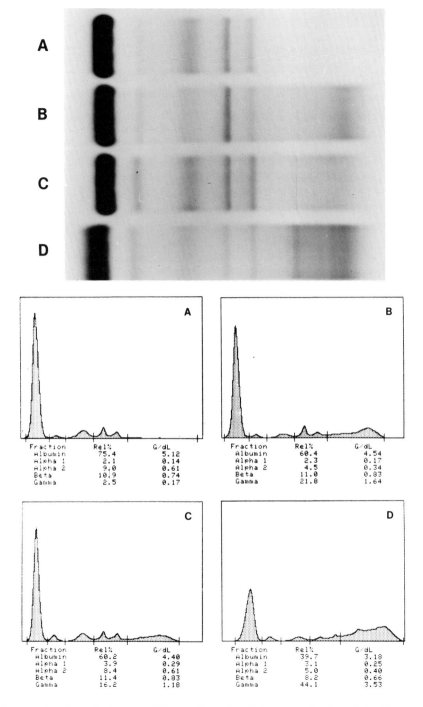

Figure 6-2. Case A: 62-year-old man. Transferred from another hospital with a need for gamma globulin replacement therapy. Case B: 74-year-old man. He had a gamma globulin level of 1.09, 6 months previously. Case C: 29-year-old woman with history of systemic lupus erythematosus. Case D: 58-year-old man.

Interpretation for Figure 6-2

Case A. There is a severe hypogammaglobulinemia. That older individuals may normally develop such deficiency is a misconception. The differential should include light chain disease, B-cell neoplasia, chemotherapy, or immune deficiency. A call to the clinician revealed that the patient had been given chemotherapy for light chain disease. His gamma globulin deficiency was so profound that he had had problems with pyogenic infections. He is now being given gamma globulin therapy for support during chemotherapy. A urine IEP was recommended both to document the light chain disease for our records and to follow the chemotherapy.

Case B. There is a broad increase in the slow gamma globulin region. Such an increase commonly occurs with hepatitis. The clinician informed us that the patient had had chronic active hepatitis, but was considered stable. The increase in gamma globulin from 6 months earlier is noted on the densitometric scan. The significance of this increase for the patient was not clear. However, a repeat electrophoresis is planned on the next 6-month visit.

Case C. There is a slight increase in the alpha-1 region. This may indicate a mild acute phase reaction, but is too nonspecific in itself for such an interpretation. Despite the history, there is no other evidence of C3 activation, increase in gamma globulin, or immune complexes.

Case D. This serum shows several abnormalities. The albumin shows an anodal slurring, which is typical of bilirubin binding but may be due to the binding of anionic drugs in other contexts. There is an increased density at the beta-gamma region, the so-called beta–gamma bridge. The gamma region is broadly increased with a few small bands that are especially prominent in the slow gamma region. This pattern has several features indicating severe liver disease. The gamma region bands probably represent immune complexes, but in this patient some may merely be oligoclonal expansion. The clinician informed me that this patient has had chronic active hepatitis for several years and recently developed ascites.

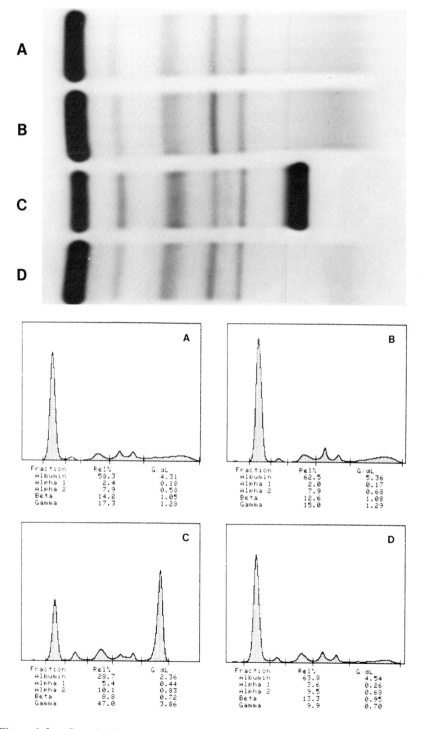

Figure 6–3. Case A: 36-year-old woman. Diabetes. Case B: 60-year-old woman. Anemia. Case C: 73-year-old man. Back strain. Case D: 66-year-old man.

Interpretations for Figure 6–3

Case A. This is a normal protein electrophoresis.

Case B. There is an increase in the transferrin band. This patient had an iron-deficiency anemia. An isolated increase in the transferrin band should at least prompt a check of the hematocrit and red cell indices.

Case C. This serum shows two ominous features. A striking fast gamma spike is obvious. Further, the remainder of the gamma globulin region is extremely faint, indicating suppression of the normal gamma globulin. The densitometry scan nicely demonstrates that the albumin is low, and an increase in both the alpha-1 and alpha-2 globulin indicates some acute phase activity. The low transferrin band is also typical of this. This patient has multiple myeloma. On calling the clinician, I was told that the patient had strained his back recently while using a ladder. He had been treated symptomatically with muscle relaxants. The serum protein electrophoresis was sent as an afterthought.

Case D. This is a normal protein electrophoresis. The gamma globulin region is in the low-normal range.

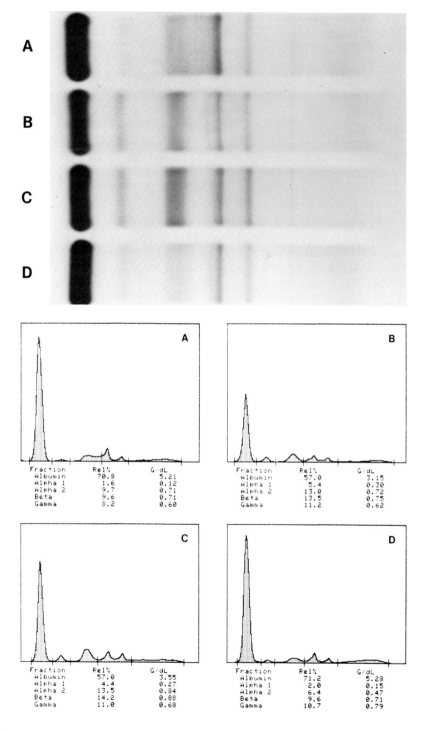

Figure 6–4. Case A: 53-year-old man. Case B: 12-year-old boy, recent infection. Case C: No information. Case D: 82-year-old woman with back pain.

Interpretations for Figure 6-4

Case A. This sample has a low-normal level of alpha-1 globulin. The most striking change is a cathodal slurring of the alpha-2 band toward the transferrin band. This type of slurring is most common with hemolysis (usually due to poor handling of the sample). On inspection of the sample, however, it was obvious that there was no hemolysis. Since prebeta lipoproteins migrate in this region, a cholesterol and triglyceride level were recommended. Triglycerides were markedly elevated with a moderate increase in cholesterol. HRE is not a test for screening lipid abnormalities. However, one must be aware that some of the changes seen may be due to lipid alterations, and appropriate subsequent testing should be recommended.

Case B. There are several abnormalities in this serum. Albumin is slightly decreased (shown best on the densitometric scan), and there is a moderate increase in the alpha-1 globulin. Alpha-2 is in the high-normal range while the transferrin band is low. C3 is low, and there is a C3c band just anodal to transferrin. Gamma globulin is in the low-normal range. This is a mild acute phase reaction pattern.

Case C. This sample has a few minor changes. The alpha-1 is slightly elevated, as is the alpha-2 and transferrin. A trivial decrease is present with the albumin. This is a nonspecific pattern. When our resident called the clinician, he found that this young woman was pregnant.

Case D. This is a normal protein electrophoresis.

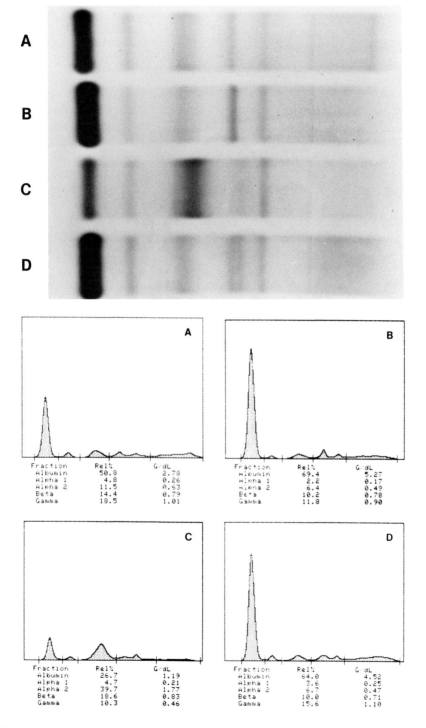

Figure 6–5. Case A: 62-year-old woman. Case B: 70-year-old man with peripheral neuropathy. Case C: 22-year-old man. Case D: 70-year-old man; rule out tertiary syphilis.

Interpretations for Figure 6-5

Case A. Two abnormalities stand out on this electrophoretic strip and the densitometric scan. The albumin is quite low (seen to best advantage on the scan) and there is a subtle area of restricted mobility (a minimonoclonal band) in the slow gamma region. Immunofixation revealed that the slow gamma band was an IgG kappa monoclonal gammopathy.

Case B. This is a normal electrophoretic pattern. Although we emphasized in Chapter 5 that peripheral neuropathy may accompany myeloma or may be related to specific binding of monoclonal proteins to myelin-associated glycoproteins, most cases of peripheral neuropathy have no such association.

Case C. This sample shows the classic nephrotic pattern. Albumin and gamma globulin are both quite low. The alpha-2 region is quite dense because of elevated alpha-2 macroglobulin. Careful examination of the area between the faintly staining transferrin band and the C3 band shows a weak, irregular band near the transferrin band; this is an elevated beta-1 lipoprotein.

Case D. This is a normal electrophoretic pattern. There is one interesting finding: The transferrin band is split into two identically staining bands. This is a transferrin variant that has no known clinical significance.

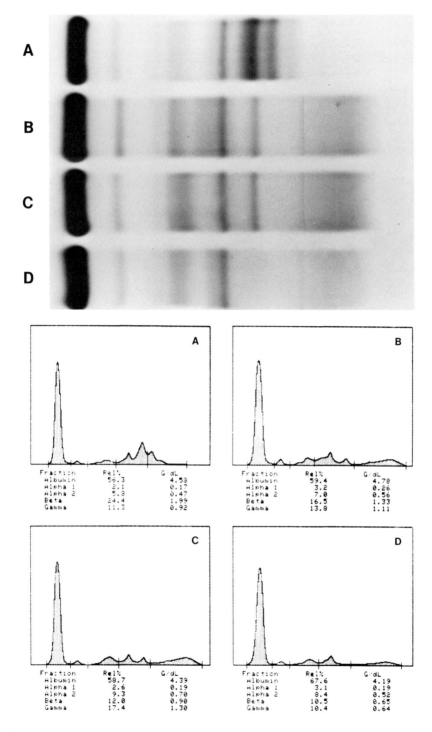

Figure 6–6. Case A: 57-year-old man, bone pain. Case B: 73-year-old woman. Case C: 40-year-old woman. Case D: No information.

197

Interpretations for Figure 6–6

Case A. This is a markedly abnormal pattern. The alpha-1 and -2 regions appear low on the strip, although this is not confirmed by the densitometric scan. The beta region is markedly abnormal, as is the gamma region on the strip. Again, the densitometric scan alone is not as impressive as the direct visualization of the electrophoretic strip. In the beta region there are three bands instead of the usual two. The most anodal is transferrin, which is normal. The darkest band is next in the usual C3 position, followed by a more weakly staining band in (approximately) the fibrinogen area. The gamma region stained abnormally lightly. Immunofixation of this sample revealed that the patient had an IgA lambda monoclonal gammopathy. Both the darkly staining band in the C3 area and the lighter staining band in the fibrinogen area were IgA lambda monoclonal proteins. The patient has multiple myeloma. It is common to find a broad band with IgA monoclonal gammopathies as the molecules tend to self-aggregate. The second, slower moving band is also not uncommon. IgA monoclonals can occur as both monomers and multimers (dimers, trimers). As stated earlier, densitometric scan quantification is not as useful in following beta-migrating monoclonal proteins because it is difficult to separate this information from the transferrin and C3 present in this region. Also, although the densitometric scan information indicates that the gamma region is a respectable 0.92 g/dl, a quick glance at the electrophoretic strip shows that there is a marked deficiency in the normal gamma globulin protein. The technologist decided to place the second monoclonal band in the gamma region, accounting for this falsely high-normal gamma region. Whenever we see such a pattern in a patient with no known file or history, we inform the clinicians about the probable myeloma.

Case B. This specimen has one subtle abnormality in the slow alpha-2 region. A hazy region merges with the transferrin band. This is a pattern often seen when specimens are hemolyzed (usually due to poor handling); this serum was hemolyzed.

Case C. This is a normal electrophoretic pattern.

Case D. Another example of our lyophilized control. The C3 band is missing and a C3c band can be seen just anodal to transferrin. The gamma region is relatively low.

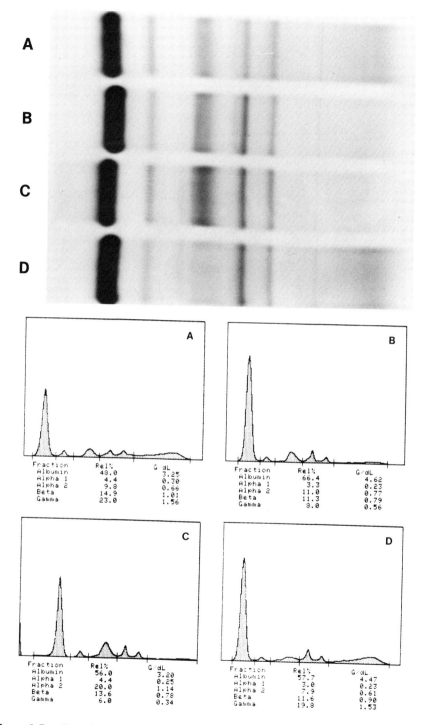

Figure 6–7. Case A: 69-year-old woman with jaundice. Case B: 6-year-old girl. Case C: 51-year-old woman with diarrhea. Case D: 36-year-old woman.

Interpretations for Figure 6–7

Case A. This serum has a few subtle abnormalities. The albumin is decreased (best seen on densitometric scan) and shows a slightly increased anodal migration. Such migration of albumin often indicates hyperbilirubinemia. The alpha-1 region is elevated and the transferrin band is slightly decreased. Together, these observations are consistent with an acute phase reaction in a jaundiced patient. There are two other findings of interest. There is a broad polyclonal increase in the gamma region, most prominently in the slow gamma region. Careful inspection of this portion of the slow gamma region reveals two fine lines separated by a clearer area, an example of the type of pattern seen with circulating immune complexes. This patient had chronic hepatitis.

Case B. This sample shows a slightly low gamma globulin region. The pediatrician was concerned about immunodeficiency disease because the child had had repeated problems with infections. Immunoglobulin quantifications revealed low-normal levels of IgG, IgA, and IgM.

Case C. This pattern has several abnormalities. There is an extremely long anodal slurring of the albumin band, which is due to heparin binding. Albumin itself is low (note the values of the densitometric scan). The alpha-1 region is in the high-normal range; there is a considerable increase in the alpha-2 region. Beta-1 lipoprotein is not elevated. The other remarkable finding is the extremely low gamma globulin region, a possible pattern from a patient with nephrotic syndrome. Indeed, the heparin effect could indicate that the patient was heparinized while on dialysis. However, the history of diarrhea and the lack of the beta-1 lipoprotein band often seen in nephrotic serum prompted a call to the clinician. The patient had normal renal function. The history was correct. For several weeks, the patient had had severe malabsorption, which was being studied. Recently, this woman developed thrombophlebitis, which required anticoagulation with heparin.

Case D. There is a diffuse increase in the gamma globulin level in this case. The alpha-2 region appears slightly low. These features are too nonspecific to render more than a descriptive report.

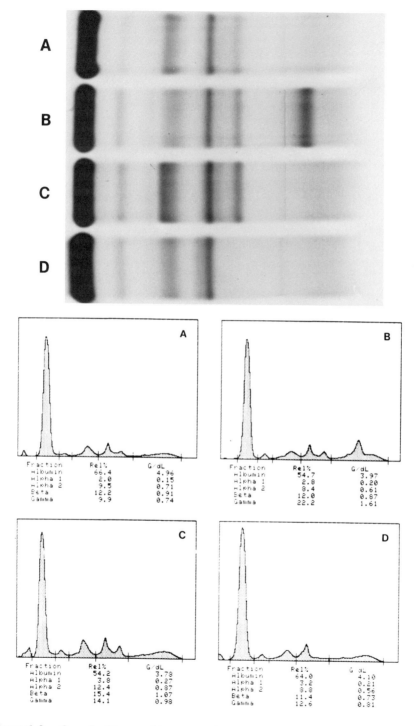

Figure 6–8. Case A: 30-year-old woman. Case B: 84-year-old woman. Case C: 24-year-old woman. Case D: Control.

Interpretations for Figure 6–8

Case A. This is a normal electrophoretic sample. The deflection anodal to albumin is an artifact. The patient's name was written on the strip too close to the albumin, and this area was scanned on all four of these cases.

Case B. A midgamma spike is the main finding. The patient has had a known IgG kappa monoclonal protein for several years. There has been no change in the electrophoretic pattern or the gamma region quantification. The sample is signed out "IgG kappa monoclonal protein persists." A noticeable increase or decrease would have been noted in the report. Note the lack of suppression of the surrounding gamma globulins, which is more typical of benign monoclonal gammopathies than of multiple myeloma. Further, the total amount of gamma protein is only modestly elevated.

Case C. This sample has elevated alpha-1, alpha-2, and transferrin. The patient was pregnant.

Case D. Once again, a lyophilized control sample (this one from Gelman) is run. It also has a C3c band anodal to the transferrin. C3 is missing.

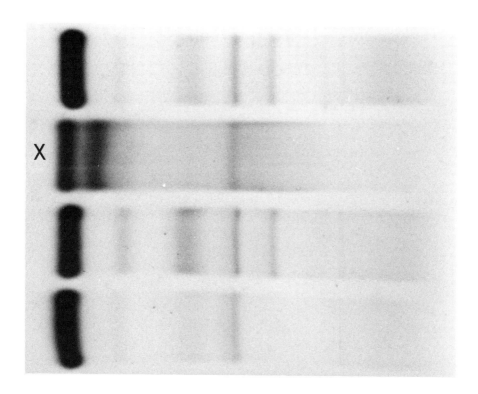

Figure 6-9. Case X: 46-year-old man, liver disease.

Interpretation for Figure 6–9

The electrophoretic pattern (X) is markedly abnormal. Two dense bands are seen in the albumin region. Although an alpha-1 antitrypsin band is not seen, one cannot be certain that the second dark albumin region band is not obscuring the alpha-1 region. There is a diffuse haze between the second albumin region band and transferrin. No distinct alpha-2 band is seen. C3 is absent although a diffuse haze extends from the transferrin band to about the origin. No staining is found in the gamma globulin region. One interpreter thought that this was a bisalbuminemia in a patient with severe liver disease. When I first saw this pattern, I doubted that it came from a human; I know of no disease that could cause such a pattern.

This is an artifact due to partial denaturation of the serum proteins. On questioning the technologist, it became clear that at the same time he was setting up his HRE patterns, he used adjacent tubes for the total protein determination (Biuret technique). We suspected that a drop of Biuret reagent may have fallen into the patient's sample. We were able to reproduce the artifact by placing a drop of Biuret reagent into the sample and performing electrophoresis. When unusual samples like this one are found and the interpretation is unclear, a repeat analysis should be done. In this case, the repeat revealed a normal electrophoretic pattern.

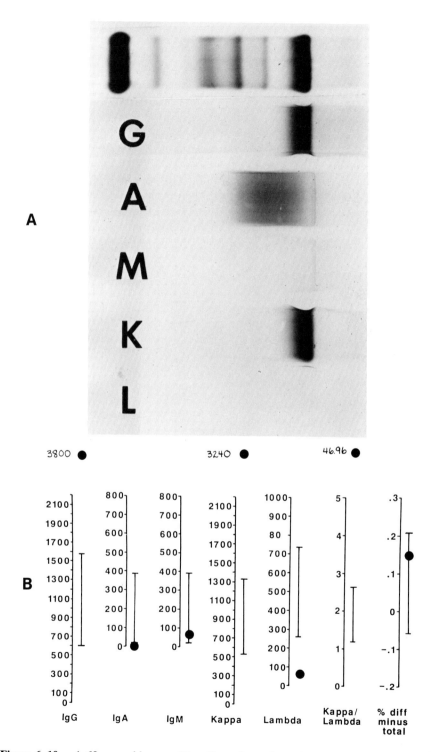

Figure 6-10. A 68-year-old man with collapsed vertebra. (Symbols: G, IgG; A, IgA; M, IgM; K, kappa; L, lambda.)

Interpretation for Figure 6–10

The HRE strip shows a large spike near the origin. The gamma region has relatively little protein. The immunofixation pattern shows an obvious IgG kappa monoclonal protein. However, it was not necessary to do the immunofixation in this case. A glance at the immunoglobulin quantifications in Figure 6–10B, together with the HRE pattern shown on the top of Figure 6–10A, already has indicated that the patient has an IgG kappa monoclonal protein. In cases such as this, we can make the diagnosis within 1 day. This shortens the workup time, and if the clinicians are awaiting this information, it can shorten the patient's hospital stay. When we find any monoclonal protein for the first time, we inform the clinician immediately, and a urine is requested to determine if the patient also has a Bence Jones protein.

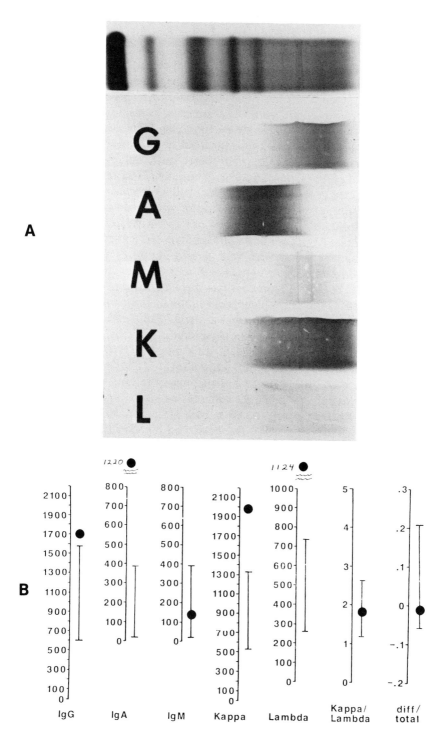

Figure 6–11. A 72-year-old woman with hip pain and anemia.

Interpretation for Figure 6–11

The HRE pattern shows increased alpha-1, alpha-2, and gamma globulins. There is a marked increase in "background" staining from the transferrin region through the end of the gamma region, which produces a striking beta-gamma bridge. This is the pattern of a patient with acute activity of a chronic inflammatory process. It is likely that a chronic process has produced a marked elevation in IgA, as this is the immunoglobulin most responsible for the beta-gamma bridge. There is no hint of any area with restricted mobility. Because of the hip pain and anemia, the clinician had requested an immunofixation. He was concerned about the possibility of the patient having myeloma. From the HRE we can see that this is a polyclonal process. The immunoglobulin quantifications shown in Figure 6–11B demonstrate the marked elevation in IgA that we suspected from the hazy beta region and strong beta–gamma bridge. The IgG is also above our upper limit of normal, consistent with the increased gamma region. IgM is in the midnormal range. Importantly, *both* kappa- and lambda-containing immunoglobulins were increased, maintaining a normal kappa/lambda ratio of 1.7. This confirms our impression that this patient has a polyclonal increase in both IgA and IgG. Uncommonly, monoclonal proteins do occur in patients with polyclonal gammopathies; however, in such cases, a distinct "M" component should be evident by HRE, which in this case it is not. Immunofixation of the sample (Figure 6–11A) is a redundant exercise that demonstrates the polyclonal nature of the process. It was not needed to make the diagnosis in this case.

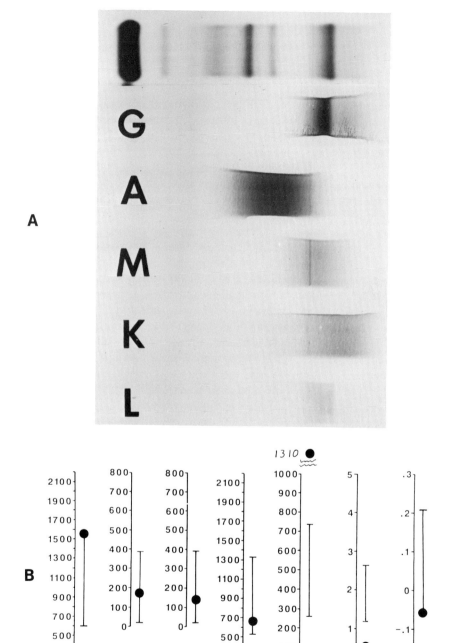

Figure 6-12. A 47-year-old man, outside sample, no history.

Interpretation for Figure 6–12

The HRE pattern shows an abnormal band in the gamma region. Note, however, that there is a diffuse haze in the gamma region. This indicates that normal IgG synthesis is not markedly suppressed, as is often true in myeloma (see Chapter 5). A band of this size in this area is going to be a monoclonal gammopathy. The immunoglobulin quantifications shown in Figure 6–12B allow us to diagnose this as an IgG lambda monoclonal gammopathy. The IgG and lambda are considerably elevated while kappa is in the low-normal range. The marked depression of the normal kappa/lambda ratio allows us to make the diagnosis. The immunofixation shown in Figure 6–12A also demonstrates the IgG lambda monoclonal gammopathy. Note that there is considerable normal IgG present, which causes the diffuse haze behind the monoclonal band and results in a kappa value in the normal range. The lambda region shows the monoclonal band in the same area as the HRE gel and the IgG immunofixation. Note, however, that it does not stain as strongly as the IgG band, which is typical for lambda-containing monoclonal proteins. Such weak staining has been known to occur in IEP, where it is often termed the "prozone" phenomenon. For this reason, one cannot judge the quantity of the protein present by the density of the band shown by either immunofixation or IEP. For quantification, we use either the densitometric estimate of the gamma region or the nephelometric measurements as shown in Figure 6–12B.

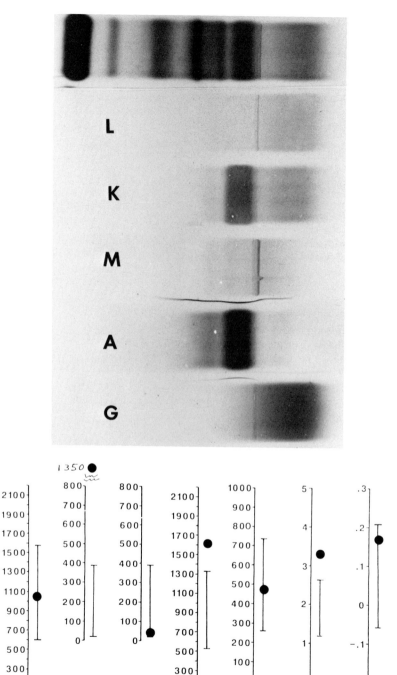

Figure 6–13. A 72-year-old woman; rule out myeloma.

Interpretation for Figure 6–13

The HRE pattern shows a very broad band in the beta–gamma region. The gamma region shows a normal, diffuse hazy area. The broad beta–gamma band is in the same area as fibrinogen. It is important to be sure that the sample is from serum. Some commercial antisera to immunoglobulins have cross-reactivity with fibrinogen, and this can confuse the interpretation of an immunofixation pattern if the sample is from plasma. In Figure 6–13B are shown the immunoglobulin quantifications for this sample. There is a marked (fivefold) increase in IgA, while IgG and IgM are in the normal and low-normal range, respectively. Kappa-containing immunoglobulins are increased and lambda-containing immunoglobulins are in the normal range; the latter is caused by the presence of the normal IgG. Nonetheless, the kappa/lambda ratio is considerably abnormal, which is typical of IgA monoclonal gammopathies. They are often broad due to self-aggregation and usually migrate in the beta or beta-gamma region. Again, the HRE and immunoglobulin quantifications together suffice to make the diagnosis. The immunofixation pattern in Figure 6–13A also demonstrates the IgA kappa monoclonal protein. Note that in the IgM reaction a dense band is present just cathodal to the origin. This is an artifact which we can see when serum is used undiluted.

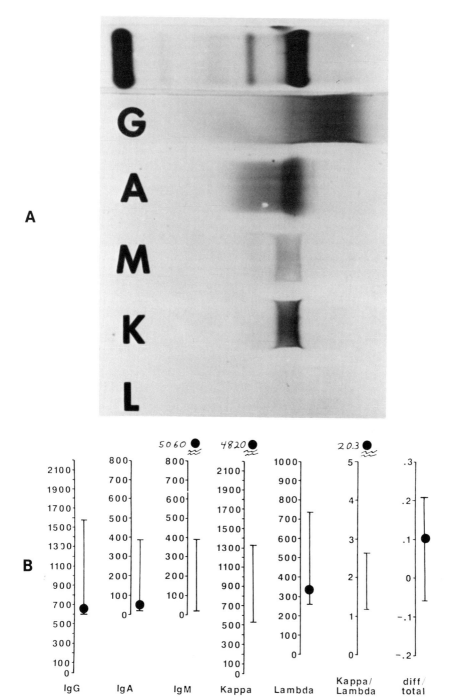

Figure 6-14. A 68-year-old woman with hyperviscosity.

Interpretation for Figure 6–14

The HRE is markedly abnormal. An enormous band is present at the origin. The alpha-1, alpha-2, and gamma regions are low. The immunoglobulin quantifications shown in Figure 6–14B clearly indicate that this is an IgM kappa monoclonal gammopathy. There is no need to perform IEP or immunofixation. Indeed, the immunofixation in Figure 6–14A is difficult to interpret. IgG is in the low-normal range (see quantification chart) and when diluted 1:6 gives a diffuse polyclonal immunofixation pattern. The IgA is very low (53 mg/dl), but on the immunofixation of the undiluted serum, a dark band is seen at the origin. This is an artifact.

The IgM monoclonal protein in this case is responsible for the hyperviscosity and tends to self-aggregate. When run undiluted, it precipitates at the origin without any antisera. The IgM reaction shows a relatively weak, broad band at the origin. The sample must be diluted 1:50 to be in the proper range for reaction. It is not clear why the reaction was so weak for this protein. The kappa shows the monoclonal band that one would expect. The serum for the lambda reaction was incorrectly diluted (1:50), so the small amount of normal lambda protein that is present was not seen. If the immunofixation was needed for diagnosis, one would repeat the lambda with the serum diluted 1:3. Fortunately, there is no reason to perform the immunofixation since the diagnosis is obvious from the immunoglobulin quantification and HRE.

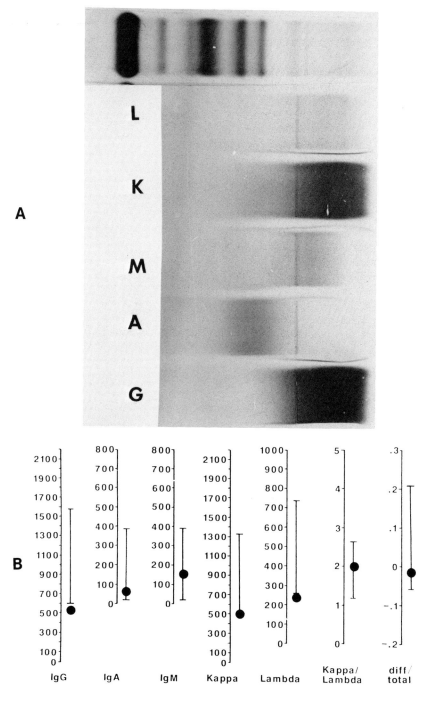

Figure 6–15. A 67-year-old woman with joint pain.

Interpretation for Figure 6–15

The HRE pattern shows a slightly low gamma region. In the midgamma region are seen two small parallel bands that are suggestive of circulating immune complexes. The immunoglobulin quantifications shown in Figure 6–15B show a slightly low IgG with normal IgA, IgM, and kappa/lambda ratio. Because of the relatively low gamma, an immunofixation was performed. IgG, IgA, and IgM are all diffusely present in their appropriate regions. However, in both the kappa and lambda reactions, two parallel bands can be seen over the background level for each of these light chains. This is typical of findings for immune complexes as they usually contain both kappa and lambda, which migrate in the same location. In this case, the HRE with the immunoglobulin quantification was insufficient to let us confidently rule out a monoclonal gammopathy. We also recommended that a urine IEP be performed to rule out light chain disease; that study was performed and was negative.

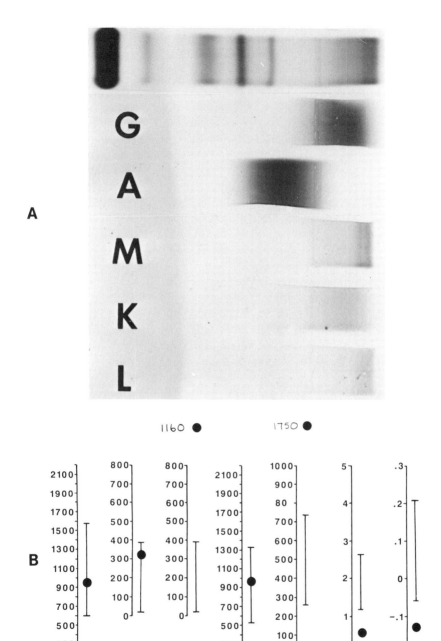

Figure 6–16. A 59-year-old man; rule out lymphoma.

Interpretation for Figure 6–16

The HRE pattern shows a diffuse gamma region with two parallel bands in the slow gamma region. We suspected that this represented circulating immune complexes. Surprisingly, the immunoglobulin quantifications in Figure 6–16B indicated that there was an IgM lambda monoclonal gammopathy. While the IgG and IgA were in the normal range, there was a marked elevation of IgM with a low kappa/lambda ratio. As this was not expected, an immunofixation was performed, confirming the impression of an IgM lambda monoclonal protein. It is unusual for IgM monoclonal proteins to migrate in the slow gamma region. Usually, IgM monoclonal proteins migrate near the origin or in the beta region. The pattern of double bands may have been due to aggregation of the IgM; however, further studies were not performed as this was peripheral to the diagnosis.

When the impression from the HRE pattern is unusual or does not fit with our expectations, we do not hesitate to confirm our impression with immunofixation. Also, if a clinician requests an immunofixation after we have formed our impression on the basis of HRE and immunoglobulin quantifications, we speak to him or her about the particular case and may run an immunofixation. In more than four years of maintaining such a policy, we have not yet found one monoclonal gammopathy. Such requests for further studies are uncommon.

Note that the diff/total was low in this case. It prompted us to perform an IEP of urine to rule out Berce Jones protein. This study was negative. We have not found the diff/total to be as useful as other parts of our strategy.

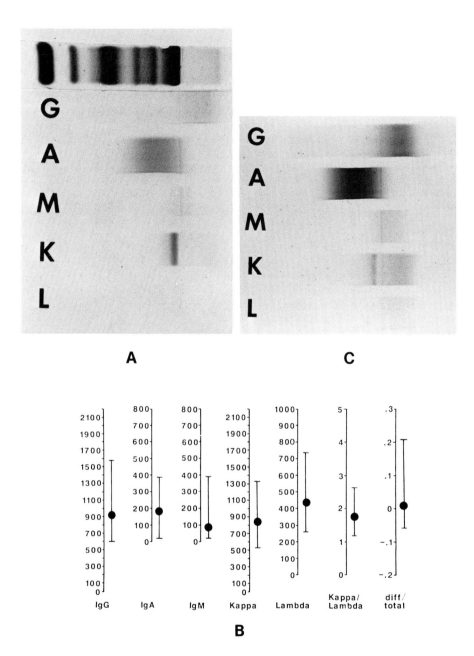

Figure 6-17. A, B. A 61-year-old man with recurrent pneumonia. Plasma sample sent from outside hospital. C. Control plasma used to test immunofixation reagents.

Interpretation for Figure 6–17

The HRE pattern shows a dense band in the beta–gamma region. Since this sample is known to be plasma, it is presumably fibrinogen. However, the immunofixation given below the electrophoresis demonstrates a band with the identical restriction, which reacts with kappa but not any of the other immunoglobulins. Quantification of the serum immunoglobulins shown in Figure 6–17A, B indicates that they are all in the normal range, including the kappa/lambda ratio. No Bence Jones protein was present in the urine. A repeat immunofixation with a serum sample that was subsequently obtained was normal. We were concerned about the new lot of antikappa which, although we had tested it against normal serum, had not been tested against plasma. Therefore, the control study with normal plasma is shown in Figure 6–17C. The same kappa band was present, indicating that that lot of antikappa had significant cross-reactivity with fibrinogen.

This case illustrates several important points. First, use serum, not plasma, for protein electrophoresis. If a real monoclonal band were present in the beta–gamma region, it would be obscured by fibrinogen. Second, when the immunoglobulin quantifications and the immunofixation do not correlate, repeat the analysis on a fresh sample to be certain that the same (correct) sample was used for both. Finally, be careful with commercial antisera preparations. Minor cross-reactivity can create problems in interpretations. Always test new antisera against your control negative serum. If you are forced to use plasma in a case, be sure to check your antisera against control plasma.

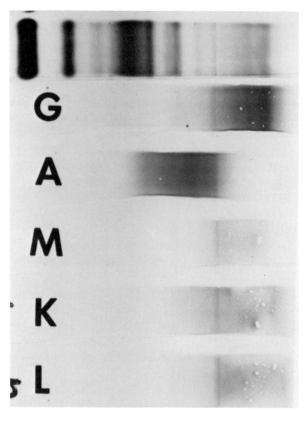

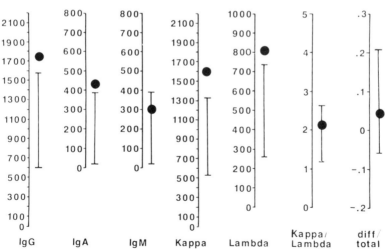

Figure 6–18. A 23-year-old man with appendicitis.

Interpretation for Figure 6-18

This sample shows an increased alpha-1 and alpha-2 globulin region. A faint band is present in the fibrinogen region indicating that the sample was not completely clotted. In the gamma region, several small bands are seen superimposed on a relatively normal gamma background. The immunoglobulin quantifications indicate that IgG and IgA are elevated with a normal IgM and kappa/lambda ratio. This is an oligoclonal expansion, which can be seen in severe acute infections such as pneumonia or, in this case, appendicitis. There is no need to perform immunofixation, which in this case shows that the oligoclonal bands were IgG. The kappa and lambda immunofixation reactions are somewhat obscured by several holes due to air-bubble artifacts. There is no evidence that a monoclonal process is present. The patient is very young, but monoclonal proteins have been found, albeit rarely, in such patients.

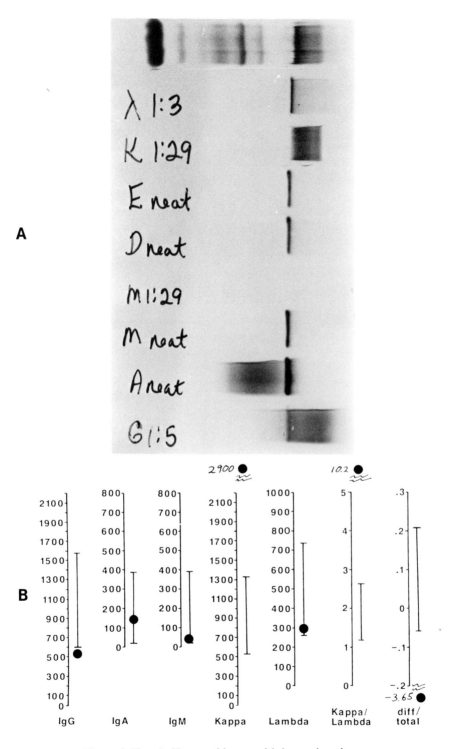

Figure 6-19. A 57-year-old man with hyperviscosity.

223

Interpretation for Figure 6-19

The HRE sample shows two remarkable features. A dense band is seen at the origin, and an extremely broad band extends into about half of the gamma globulin region where it stops abruptly. The immunoglobulin quantifications shown in Figure 6-19B indicate that the IgG is below our lower limit of normal; IgM is relatively low and IgA is normal. The kappa/lambda ratio is markedly elevated due to the extraordinary increase in kappa chains. This appears to be kappa light chain disease, but such a large band in the serum is unusual; usually, these proteins pass into the urine. The history of hyperviscosity causes one to think of Waldenstrom's macroglobulinemia, but the IgM is quite low.

Because of these findings, the immunofixation in Figure 6-19A included antibodies to IgE and IgD to see if they were bound to the peculiar kappa chain. The extremely dense band at the origin is present in all, except in the kappa and IgM reactions in which the serum was diluted 1:29. This indicates that the abnormal band is precipitating at the origin, due to self-aggregation like a cryoglobulin. At the more dilute concentration of 1:29, the aggregation is not seen. IgM was run on undiluted serum and on serum diluted 1:29, because the history of hyperviscosity suggested Waldenstrom's macroglobulinemia and we were concerned that the nephelometer may have missed the IgM despite our antigen excess check. We were wrong. The instrument correctly quantified the IgM. The other remarkable feature of the immunofixation pattern is that the kappa reaction exactly parallels the broad dense band that extends into the gamma region and then stops abruptly. No such band is seen in the lambda reaction. The lack of reactivity in the IgD or IgE, both of which show the artifact of the monoclonal protein precipitated at the origin, gives us the diagnosis of kappa light chain disease. Urine was strongly positive for Bence Jones protein.

Light chain disease with hyperviscosity is extremely rare. The kappa light chains in this case could be broken by reducing the disulfide bonds with either 2-mercaptoethanol or dithiothreitol. The molecular weight of the unreduced molecule was greater than 600,000. On plasmapheresis therapy, the patient has improved.

One other feature to note in this case is the last column in the immunoglobulin quantification chart (Figure 6-19B). This column shows:

$$\frac{(\text{IgG} + \text{IgA} + \text{IgM}) - (\text{kappa} + \text{lambda})}{(\text{IgG} + \text{IgA} + \text{IgM})}$$

In cases of light chain disease, there can be considerably more kappa or lambda than intact immunoglobulins. This is especially true in cases of tetrameric kappa chain disease, or self-aggregating kappa chains, as in the present case. Therefore, when the light chains are subtracted from the total intact immunoglobulins, a large negative number will be obtained. After dividing by the total immunoglobulins, this gives a negative number on the "diff/total" column. From this chart, our strong initial suspicion was that this man had a strange form of kappa light chain disease. The immunofixation and reduction studies helped confirm this impression.

GENERAL COMMENTS ABOUT INTERPRETATION

The combined use of HRE and immunoglobulin quantification allows us to make the diagnosis of monoclonal gammopathy without any further serum studies in most cases. When at all unsure about a diagnosis, we resort to immunofixation, which usually confirms our impression. Caution is needed when small monoclonal bands are seen in the HRE pattern. These will usually not cause an alteration in the normal kappa/lambda ratio; they may be small monoclonal gammopathies, part of an oligoclonal expansion associated with infection or autoimmune disease, or another protein (fibrinogen in poorly clotted serum, C-reactive protein in a strong acute phase reaction). If the immunofixation shows one monoclonal band, the clinician is contacted to correlate our findings with the clinical picture. When the patient has no evidence of a neoplastic process, we recommend a urine for Bence Jones protein and a repeat of HRE in 6–12 months to see if the monoclonal protein is in fact an unusual response to infection or some other stimulation. If it persists, the patient is assumed to have a monoclonal expansion along the B-cell lineage and should be followed for this. Many such processes will pursue a benign course, but we cannot yet predict with confidence which these will be; others will develop the numerous conditions discussed in Chapter 5.

The combined use of high-resolution electrophoresis, immunoglobulin quantification, and immunofixation allows us to detect many clinically significant protein abnormalities and quickly determine the presence of monoclonal gammopathies. Special techniques, such as 2-mercaptoethanol treatment of samples and column chromatography, are only rarely used. The major caution with immunofixation is to use the proper dilution of the patient's serum and to be careful about minor reactivities with commercial antisera. If a suspected monoclonal band lines up with transferrin, C3, or fibrinogen, be sure you have checked the reactivity of that commercial antisera against those same proteins in a control sample. Finally, when the finding is new (not known from the given history or your records) or does not fit with the clinical information, review the case with the clinician.

INDEX

iron-refractory, 44
transferrin concentrations in, 44
Angioimmunoblastic lymphadenopathy,
  monoclonal proteins in, 159
Appendicitis, 221 (figure), 222
Appendix, and B lymphocytes, 132
Autoimmune disease
  differential diagnosis of, 20
  haptoglobulin increases in, 39–40
  immunoglobulin A (IgA) in, 59
  immunoglobulin G (IgG) in, 58
  serum pattern diagnosis and, 82–83
  urine pattern analysis and, 95

Bence Jones proteins (BJP)
  amyloidosis with, 161
  findings often mistaken for, 95 (fig-
    ure), 96 (figure)
  heat precipitation test of urine in,
    142–143
  high-resolution electrophoresis of, 45,
    46
  immunoelectrophoresis (IEP) and,
    114, 116 (figure)
  light chain disease with, 141, 142–143,
    145, 176
  monoclonal gammopathy diagnosis
    and, 169, 175, 176
  multiple myeloma and, 8, 20, 137,
    141
  renal disease and, 99–100
  serum protein binding by, 145, 148
    (figure)
  urine pattern analysis and, 94, 95 (fig-
    ure), 96 (figure), 145
  zone electrophoresis of, 8–9
Beta-gamma bridging
  case studies with, 189 (figure), 190,
    207 (figure), 208
  cirrhosis and, 73, 74
Beta globulin
  densitometric scan-eluted protein con-
    centration comparison for, 6
  endosmosis and migration of, 5
  high-resolution electrophoresis densi-
    tometry-cellulose acetate compari-
    son for, 17–18
  liver disease and, 7
  moving boundary electrophoresis
    with, 4
Beta lipoprotein
  agar gel absorption of, 6

cirrhosis and, 74
high-resolution electrophoresis of, 46,
  47 (figure)
nephrotic syndrome and, 77, 78
Beta-migrating monoclonal gammopathies, and transferrin, 45, 69–70
Beta-2 microglobulin
  renal disease with, 97, 98
  urine pattern analysis and, 93, 94
Biclonal gammopathies, 150–152, 151
  (figure)
  B-lymphocyte development and, 133
  immunoelectrophoresis (IEP) and, 117
  immunofixation and, 121, 123 (figure)
  reasons for occurrence of, 151–152
  use of term, 150
Biliary obstruction, serum pattern diagnosis of, 76
Bilirubin
  biliary obstruction and, 76
  cirrhosis and, 73
  hepatitis and, 75
Birth control pills. See Contraceptive
  drugs
Bisalbuminemia, 29
B lymphocytes
  activation of, 134
  chronic lymphocytic leukemia with,
    7–8
  immunoglobulin D (IgD) and, 60
  monoclonal gammopathy of undeter-
    mined significance and, 162
  multiple myeloma and, 138
  ontogeny of, 131–134
  origin of name, 132
B-lymphocyte neoplasms
  high-resolution electrophoresis in, 20,
    21
  monoclonal gammopathies in,
    157–167
  small monoclonal bands in, 20, 21
Bone marrow
  B-lymphocyte development and, 132
  multiple myeloma and, 137, 138
  T-lymphocyte development and, 134
  Waldenstrom's macroglobulinemia
    and, 154
Bovidae proteins, and immunofixation,
  127–128
Bruton's x-linked agammaglobulinemia,
  8, 131
Burkitt's lymphoma, monoclonal gammopathies in, 119, 159
Bursa of Fabricius, 132